Preventive *chemotherapy* in human helminthiasis

Coordinated use of anthelminthic drugs in control interventions:

a manual for health professionals and programme managers

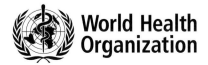
World Health Organization

WHO Library Cataloguing-in-Publication Data

Preventive chemotherapy in human helminthiasis : coordinated use of anthelminthic drugs in control interventions : a manual for health professionals and programme managers.

"A first draft of this manual was prepared by the World Health Organization (WHO) in consultation with Professor D. W. T. Crompton…"--Preface.

1.Helminthiasis - prevention and control. 2.Helminthiasis - drug therapy. 3.Anthelmintics - administration and dosage. 4.Manuals. I.Crompton, D. W. T. II.World Health Organization.

ISBN 92 4 154710 3   (NLM classification: WC 800)
ISBN 978 92 4 154710 9

Preventive Chemotherapy and Transmission Control (PCT)
Department of Control of Neglected Tropical Diseases (NTD)
World Health Organization
20, Avenue Appia
1211 Geneva 27, Switzerland

Contents

Acknowledgements

The World Health Organization (WHO) would like to express special thanks to Professor D. W. T. Crompton, University of Glasgow, Scotland, for his major contribution to the development of this manual.

The writing committee was made up of Dr Marco Albonico, Ivo de Carneri Foundation, Italy, Professor Nilanthi de Silva, University of Kelaniya Ragama, Sri Lanka, and Dr Dirk Engels, Dr Albis Francesco Gabrielli, Dr Francesco Rio and Dr Lorenzo Savioli, WHO.

Thanks are due to Ms Henrietta Allen, Dr Uche V. Amazigo, Dr Steven K. Ault, Dr Ousmane Bangoura, Dr Gautam Biswas, Dr Boakye Boatin, Dr Loretta Brabin, Dr Mark Bradley, Dr Gabriele Braeunlich, Dr Pierre Brantus, Dr Lester Chitsulo, Ms Brenda D. Colatrella, Dr Ian Darnton-Hill, Dr Denis Daumerie, Dr Michael S. Deming, Dr Mark L. Eberhard, Dr John Ehrenberg, Dr Francisco Espejo, Professor Alan Fenwick, Dr Reinhard Fescharek, Dr Justine Frain, Dr Ana Gupta, Dr Theresa Gyorkos, Dr Zoheir Hallaj, Dr Ralph H. Henderson, Dr Suzanne Hill, Dr Hans V. Hogerzeil, Professor Moazzem Hossain, Professor Peter J. Hotez, Dr Narcis B. Kabatereine, Dr Jacob Kumaresan, Dr Dominique Kyelem, Dr Patrick Lammie, Dr Janis K. Lazdins-Helds, Dr William Lin, Dr Derek Lobo, Dr Paula Luff, Dr Silvio Mariotti, Dr Matthews Mathai, Professor David Molyneux, Dr Antonio Montresor, Dr Likezo Mubila, Dr Kopano Mukelabai, Dr James N. Mwanzia, Dr Oscar Noya-González, Dr Annette Olsen, Dr Niels Ørnbjerg, Dr Eric A. Ottesen, Dr Kevin Palmer, Dr Frank Richards, Dr Robert G. Ridley, Dr Michael Schoettler, Dr Martin Springsklee, Dr Bjørn Thylefors, Dr Nana Twum-Danso, Mr Andy L. D. Wright and Dr Concepción Zuniga Valeriano for their contributions, suggestions and support and to Mrs Sarah Ballance for the technical editing of the manual.

Grateful acknowledgement is also extended to the Bill & Melinda Gates Foundation for its financial assistance with the publishing of this document.

The cover design was kindly provided by Professor D. W. T. Crompton and is based on an image from *National Geographic* magazine.

Abbreviations

ALB	albendazole
APOC	African Programme for Onchocerciasis Control
CDTI	community-directed treatment with ivermectin
DEC	diethylcarbamazine (citrate)
EPI	Expanded Programme on Immunization
GLP	good laboratory practice
GMP	good manufacturing practice
IVM	ivermectin
LEV	levamisole
LF	lymphatic filariasis
MBD	mebendazole
MDA	mass drug administration
NGDO	nongovernmental development organization
NGO	nongovernmental organization
ONCHO	onchocerciasis
PPC	Partners for Parasite Control
PYR	pyrantel
PZQ	praziquantel
SAE	serious adverse experience
SCH	schistosomiasis
SCHi	intestinal schistosomiasis
SCHu	urinary schistosomiasis
STH	soil-transmitted helminthiasis

Preface

A first draft of this manual was prepared by the World Health Organization (WHO) in consultation with Professor D.W.T. Crompton, Institute of Biomedical and Life Sciences, University of Glasgow, Scotland.

After circulation to a number of experts, the draft was revised in the light of their comments and input. It was further reviewed at the Informal Consultation on Preventive Chemotherapy in Human Helminthiasis, which took place at WHO headquarters in Geneva, Switzerland, on 16–17 March 2006.

Subsequently, WHO staff, in close collaboration with Professor D.W.T. Crompton, who chaired the Informal Consultation, undertook further revision of the manual on the basis of comments and suggestions made by participants. The resulting draft was circulated to all concerned before being finalized for publication.

Glossary

The definitions given below apply to the terms as used in this manual. They may have different meanings in other contexts.

adverse reaction (to a drug)
Noxious and unintended reaction, which occurs at doses normally used in humans for the prophylaxis, diagnosis or treatment of disease, or for the modification of physiological function.

drug distribution channel
The mechanism through which anthelminthic drugs are provided to target communities or population groups.

eligible population
Group of individuals qualified or entitled to receive anthelminthic treatment in preventive chemotherapy interventions. Eligible populations may vary from high-risk groups in targeted treatment interventions to the entire population living in endemic areas in mass drug administration (MDA) interventions. See also *ineligible population*.

haematuria
Presence of red blood cells in the urine.
Macrohaematuria – blood is present in sufficient quantity to be seen by visual inspection of the urine sample (the urine is red or brown in colour).
Microhaematuria – blood is present in insufficient quantity to be visible to the naked eye but is detectable using a reagent strip.

helminthiasis
A general term for any form of disease that accompanies a helminth infection. In most cases the onset and severity of detectable morbidity in a person are related to the number of worms present.

hydrocele
Collection of fluid in the scrotal sac around the testicles. Usually painless, it is a common chronic manifestation of lymphatic filariasis.

ineligible population
Group of individuals not qualified or entitled to receive anthelminthic treatment in preventive chemotherapy interventions. Ineligibility is usually determined by exclusion criteria based on drug safety.

lymphoedema
Swelling of a body part (usually limbs, breast or genitals) caused by blockage of, or damage to, the drainage of the lymphatic system. It is a chronic manifestation of lymphatic filariasis.

mass drug administration (MDA)
Distribution of drugs to the entire population of a given administrative setting (state, region, province, district, sub-district, village, etc.); however, exclusion criteria may apply (see *ineligible population*). MDA entails close collaboration between the organization responsible for drug distribution (usually the ministry of health) and target communities: if MDA is undertaken under the direction of the community itself, the term community-directed treatment (ComDT) may also be used. The main application of the ComDT approach has been to onchocerciasis control, and community-directed treatment with ivermectin (CDTI) is the principal strategy adopted by the African Programme for Onchocerciasis Control (APOC).

MDA is a public health intervention that can be implemented through a number of different approaches:

House-to-house administration (*mobile teams*). The drug distributor collects the drug from a designated centre and goes from house to house to administer it. This approach ensures coverage of all households but is labour-intensive, especially in areas where population density is low and household members may be away from home during the time of drug distribution.

Booth distribution (*fixed teams*). Drug distribution booths are set up at sites selected to be accessible to the community. Drug distributors administer the drugs to the beneficiaries who come to the booth. This approach is suitable in urban situations, but coverage depends on the motivation of the beneficiaries. Supplying the booths with drugs and potable water for swallowing the drugs is logistically demanding.

Administering drugs in special population groups. Certain population groups can easily be reached at particular locations: students in schools, patients in hospitals, workers at commercial establishments, major building sites and industrial sites, inmates in prisons, and displaced persons in refugee camps.

Areas of community gatherings. Marketplaces, bus and railway stations, fairs and festivals, places of worship, and other sites where people congregate can also be used to reach the community.

With an intensive campaign approach, MDA may be organized as a national day or over a week. However, if logistic constraints make such a focused approach impracticable, the distribution could be staggered over a period of 3–4 weeks.

morbidity
Detectable and measurable consequences of a disease. Evidence of morbidity due to helminthic diseases may be overt (such as the presence of blood in the urine, anaemia, chronic pain or fatigue) or subtle (such as stunted growth, impeded school or work performance or increased susceptibility to other diseases).

preschool children

All children between the ages of 1 and 5 years who are not yet attending (primary) school.

prevalence of infection

The proportion of individuals in a population infected with a specified agent.

prevalence of any infection

The proportion of individuals in a population infected with at least one agent. The concept is used for appropriate community diagnosis in soil-transmitted helminthiasis: proportion of individuals in a population infected with at least one soil-transmitted helminth species (*Ascaris lumbricoides, Trichuris trichiura, Ancylostoma duodenale, Necator americanus*).

preventive (anthelminthic) chemotherapy

Use of anthelminthic drugs, either alone or in combination, as a public health tool against helminth infections.

RAPLOA

A rapid assessment procedure for *Loa loa*, which uses a simple questionnaire on the history of eye worm (i.e. eye worm lasting less than 7 days and confirmed by a photograph of an adult *L. loa* worm in the eye) to predict whether or not loiasis is present in a community at a high level of endemicity.

SAFE

A strategy that consists of lid surgery (S), antibiotics to treat the community pool of infection (A), facial cleanliness (F), and environmental changes (E).

school-age children

All children between the ages of 6 and 15 years (usually), regardless of whether they are attending school. In some countries, a primary school's enrolment may include individuals older than 15 years.

serious adverse experience (SAE)

An event that is fatal, life-threatening, disabling, or incapacitating or that results in hospitalization after drug intake. Any experience that the investigator regards as serious or that would suggest any significant hazard, contraindication, side-effect, or precaution that may be associated with the use of the drug should be reported. See Annex 3 for a standardized form for recording SAE.

targeted treatment

Group-level application of anthelminthic drugs where the group eligible for treatment may be defined by age, sex, or other social characteristics irrespective of infection status (exclusion criteria may apply).

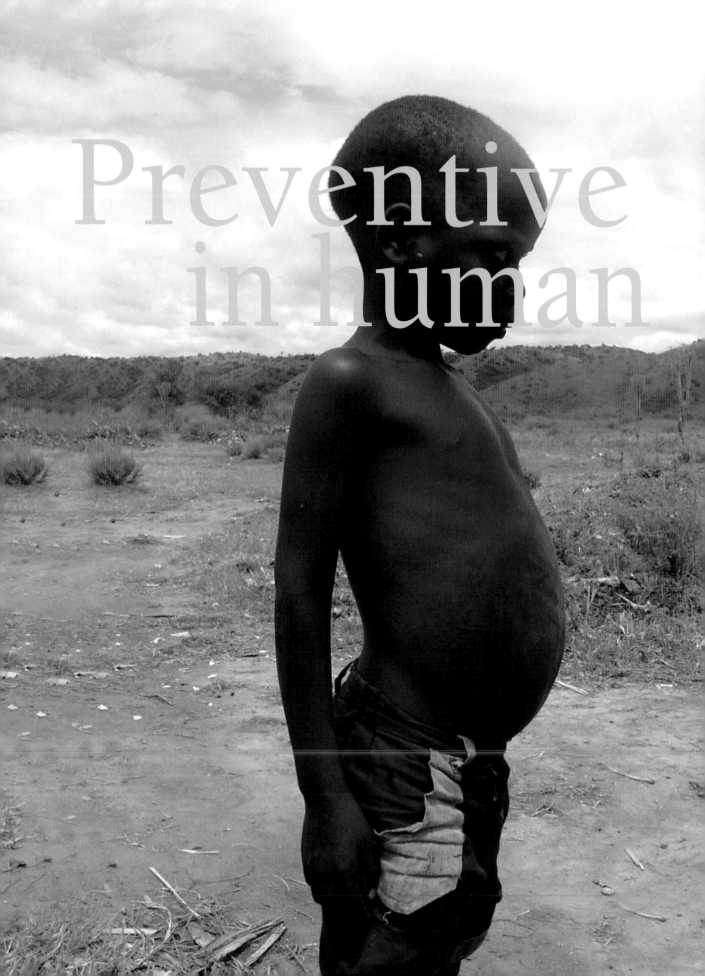

chemotherapy
helminthiasis

1. MEETING THE CHALLENGE

Helminth infections impose a great burden on poor populations in the developing world – yet robust, low-cost and effective public health interventions are available to relieve that burden and provide a better quality of life for people in poor settings.

Control of disease due to helminth infections, as well as to other agents, aims to alleviate suffering, reduce poverty, and support equal opportunities for men and women. Preventive chemotherapy uses the available anthelminthic drugs – either alone or in combination – as a public health tool for preventing morbidity due to infection usually with more than one helminth at a time; in certain epidemiological conditions contributes also to sustained reduction of transmission. Since many of these drugs are broad-spectrum, allowing several diseases to be tackled simultaneously, preventive chemotherapy interventions should be conceived as drug-based rather than disease-based: emphasis should be on the best, coordinated use of the available drugs rather than on specific forms of helminthiasis.

Although chemotherapy of human helminthiasis is the focus of this manual, there is huge potential for its integration with the treatment of other diseases. For example, trachoma[1] control through the SAFE strategy – combining drug treatment with hygiene and environmental management – can be linked to helminth control interventions to improve the overall health of affected communities.

The greatest challenge is to extend regular anthelminthic drug coverage as a public health intervention to reach all individuals at risk of the morbidity caused by helminthic infections. Preventive chemotherapy

... emphasis should be on the best, coordinated use of the available drugs rather than on specific forms of helminthiasis.

The greatest challenge is to extend regular anthelminthic drug coverage as a public health intervention to reach all individuals at risk of the morbidity caused by helminthic infections.

[1] Trachoma is an eye infection caused by *Chlamydia trachomatis*, which may result in chronic scarring and blindness if left untreated.

should therefore begin early in life, and every opportunity should be taken to reach at-risk populations. This manual advocates much greater coordination among disease control interventions than has hitherto been seen as specific – and therefore implemented separately. Because such large numbers of people are affected, and are often difficult to reach, it also stresses the need to make the best use of all existing drug distribution channels to deliver anthelminthic drugs, and aims at encouraging programme managers to find other innovative means of reaching those in need in a sustainable manner. The result will be gains in the health, education, economic status and social well-being of entire populations. Such advances will help to build a solid foundation for improvements in maternal health and the development of children into adults free of the burden of disabling disease.

Reducing the burden of morbidity and impaired development that characterizes human helminthiasis depends on policy decisions taken by ministers of health, ministers of education and their advisers. Critically, it will depend also on the dedication of health professionals and the support of partners who have committed time, money and resources to helminth control and the involvement of communities.

This manual is intended to guide the coordinated implementation of regular, systematic, large-scale interventions that provide anthelminthic drug treatment as a core component of the joint and synergic control of helminthic diseases such as lymphatic filariasis, onchocerciasis, schistosomiasis and soil-transmitted helminthiasis. While it is a general document, intended to be applicable in all epidemiological situations, it is specific in that it deals only with drugs and their coordinated use: it does not cover any of the other important public health interventions – health education, sanitation, safe water supply, vector control, etc. – needed to ensure sustained reduction in transmission, and then elimination, of helminthiasis. It will be the responsibility of programme managers to adapt this manual to the prevailing regional, national and local context and the resources available, and to build the preventive chemotherapy component into more comprehensive control or elimination strategies already in place or planned for the future.

2. SITUATION ANALYSIS

The epidemiological distribution of lymphatic filariasis and onchocerciasis is well known. Mapping of lymphatic filariasis is almost complete in the more than 80 countries where the disease is endemic. Onchocerciasis has been thoroughly mapped, both in Africa and in the Americas. In Africa, mapping the distribution of loiasis (infection with *Loa loa*) is also important because this disease has implications for large-scale preventive chemotherapy interventions using ivermectin.

The distribution of schistosomiasis and soil-transmitted helminthiasis is less well mapped on a worldwide scale. Soil-transmitted helminthiasis is widespread in most poverty-stricken areas in the developing world; schistosomiasis occurs in focal pockets and is closely linked to the presence of water bodies that harbour susceptible species of snails.

Countries where lymphatic filariasis, onchocerciasis, schistosomiasis, soil-transmitted helminthiasis and loiasis are endemic and likely to require preventive chemotherapy are listed in Annex 1. Annex 6 lists web sites where updated information on the epidemiological distribution of each helminth infection can be found.

Simple tools and methods exist for assessing the presence and endemicity at the district level of both soil-transmitted helminthiasis and the different forms of schistosomiasis (Annex 2). It is particularly important that programme managers carry out a detailed geographical assessment of schistosomiasis in order to focus the use of praziquantel to the areas in real need, since it is the most expensive (US$ 0.08 per 600-mg tablet or US$ 0.20–0.30 per average dose) of the anthelminthic drugs available for large-scale use.

3. PREVENTIVE CHEMOTHERAPY AND ITS ROLE IN THE CONTROL OF HELMINTHIASIS

3.1 Aim and rationale

The aim of preventive chemotherapy is to avert the widespread morbidity that invariably accompanies helminth and other infections – and sometimes leads to death. Early and regular administration of the anthelminthic drugs recommended by WHO reduces the occurrence, extent, severity and long-term consequences of morbidity, and in certain epidemiological conditions contributes to sustained reduction in transmission. In practice, preventive chemotherapy requires the delivery of good-quality drugs, either alone or in combination, to as many people in need as possible at regular intervals throughout their lives: high priority should be given to achieving full coverage of targeted risk groups.

Rather than identifying every infected individual, large-scale preventive chemotherapy interventions assess entire communities for endemicity or ongoing transmission of the target helminthic diseases. The recommended drug or drug combination is then administered to all eligible members of the endemic communities. Extensive experience of the use of anthelminthic drugs has shown them to have excellent safety records, regardless of infection status; it is this safety that is key to large-scale interventions, particularly when individual diagnostic methods may be impossible to implement.

Preventive chemotherapy is perceived by both the scientific community and affected populations as an urgent need; as a public health intervention that targets the poorest sectors of humanity, anthelminthic treatment should be provided free of charge.

Box A. The role of social mobilization

Large-scale preventive chemotherapy targets all eligible individuals in communities identified as endemic for the target disease. Every individual is considered to be at risk of the disease and its sequelae. Because helminth diseases do not rapidly cause death and are more insidious in nature than many diseases of acute onset, they are rarely given priority by health providers.

The objective of preventive chemotherapy interventions is to ensure that all eligible individuals in at-risk communities swallow the recommended drugs. This behavioural change is dependent on the motivation of the at-risk individual to accept treatment as well as on the health-care provider or community volunteer adequately informing and motivating the community. Social mobilization is a complex process – the programme, health-care delivery services, health-care providers and strategies for mobilization and communication interact to influence and change the behaviour of the people. Experiences with existing health-care programmes have shown that this aspect of social mobilization, though important, is not given adequate priority during planning of preventive chemotherapy interventions (1). As community characteristics and responses to various communications from the health-care providers are different, a proper understanding of these is essential in planning effective social mobilization campaigns. Programme managers are advised to seek the assistance of social scientists and communication experts in planning and evaluating such strategies. Investment in social mobilization strategies is critical to sustaining high drug coverage throughout the duration of the programme.

Initially, preventive chemotherapy will be directed against the following four common forms of helminthiasis, which are:

- Lymphatic filariasis (LF) – caused by infection with the nematodes *Wuchereria bancrofti, Brugia malayi* and *B. timori*.

- Onchocerciasis (ONCHO) – caused by infection with the nematode *Onchocerca volvulus*.

- Schistosomiasis (SCH) – SCHi (intestinal schistosomiasis) caused by infection with the trematodes *Schistosoma mansoni, S. mekongi, S. japonicum* and *S. intercalatum*, and SCHu (urinary schistosomiasis) caused by infection with *S. haematobium*.

- Soil-transmitted helminthiasis (STH) – caused by infection with the nematodes *Ascaris lumbricoides* (roundworm), *Ancylostoma duodenale* and *Necator americanus* (hookworm), and *Trichuris trichiura* (whipworm).

Morbidity refers to the detectable and measurable signs and symptoms of a disease. Overt morbidity due to helminthiasis includes: acute adenolymphangitis, lymphoedema, hydrocele, renal disorders and chyluria (LF); skin and eye lesions (ONCHO); intestinal damage and pathological changes in the liver, eventually leading to portal hypertension (SCHi); pathological changes in kidney and bladder, and lesions caused by schistosome eggs in the genital tract, especially in women (female genital schistosomiasis) (SCHu); iron-deficiency anaemia, micronutrient deficiencies, growth retardation and intestinal obstruction (STH) (*2*). Further details on morbidity due to helminthic diseases are provided in Annex 6.

Evidence indicates that children acquire helminth infections early in life. Early infection causes initial organ damage that can remain subclinical for years and manifest overtly only later, in adulthood (*3–6*).

Organ pathology specific for each form of helminthiasis is flanked by subtle morbidity that includes impaired cognitive performance, chronic fatigue and unremitting pain, all conditions leading to increased school absenteeism, reduced worker productivity, lowered self-esteem, and social exclusion (*7–9*). Evidence is emerging to suggest that helminthiasis also exacerbates the transmission and/or severity of HIV/AIDS, malaria and tuberculosis (*10–12*). Although the annual death rate from helminthiasis is low relative to the millions of cases, helminth infections should not be neglected – they constitute a large burden on human health and resources.

More types of helminth infection than are covered in this manual will be addressed as preventive chemotherapy develops. Affected populations are urgently in need of regular treatment for other helminthiases, such as food-borne trematodiasis (clonorchiasis, opisthorchiasis, paragonimiasis and fascioliasis). Although these diseases can be treated with the same group of drugs, more evidence is needed about the impact of the drugs on morbidity before treatment schedules can be recommended. Morbidity in cestodiasis (alveolar and cystic echinococcosis, and neurocysticercosis) can be prevented by providing anthelminthic treatment for infected definitive or intermediate hosts (either humans or domestic animals that share the human environment). Operational research must be extended to develop treatment strategies for strongyloidiasis. Information about WHO-recommended anthelminthic drugs and their target diseases is summarized in Table 1.

Table 1. WHO-recommended anthelminthic drugs for use in preventive chemotherapy[a,b]

Note: Drug names are given in full in the list of abbreviations at the front of the manual.

	Disease	ALB	MBD	DEC	IVM	PZQ	LEV[c]	PYR[c]
Target diseases for which a well-defined strategy is available	Ascariasis	✓	✓	–	(✓)	–	✓	✓
	Hookworm disease	✓	✓	–	–	–	✓	✓
	Lymphatic filariasis	✓	–	✓	✓	–	–	–
	Onchocerciasis	–	–	–	✓	–	–	–
	Schistosomiasis	–	–	–	–	✓	–	–
	Trichuriasis	✓	✓	–	(✓)	–	(✓)[d]	(✓)[d]
Target diseases for which a strategy is being developed	Clonorchiasis	–	–	–	–	✓	–	–
	Opisthorchiasis	–	–	–	–	✓	–	–
	Paragonimiasis	–	–	–	–	✓	–	–
	Strongyloidiasis	✓	(✓)	–	✓	–	–	–
	Taeniasis	–	–	–	–	✓ (up to 10 mg/kg)	–	–
	Cutaneous larva migrans (zoonotic ancylostomiasis)	✓	(✓)	–	(✓)	–	(✓)	(✓)
Additional benefits	Ectoparasitic infections (scabies and lice)	–	–	–	✓	–	–	–
	Enterobiasis	✓	✓	–	(✓)	–	(✓)	✓
	Intestinal trematodiases	–	–	–	–	✓	–	–
	Visceral larva migrans (toxocariasis)	–	–	✓	(✓)	–	–	–

[a] Prescribing information and contraindications are given in the *WHO Model Formulary 2004 (13)*.

[b] In this table, ✓ indicates drugs recommended by WHO for treatment of the relevant disease, and (✓) indicates drugs that are not recommended for treatment but that have a (suboptimal) effect against the disease.

[c] At present, LEV and PYR do not have a prominent role in preventive chemotherapy as described in this manual. However, they remain useful drugs for the treatment of soil-transmitted helminthiasis, and since – unlike ALB and MBD – they do not belong to the benzimidazole group, they will be expected to contribute to the management of drug-resistant STH infections should that problem emerge.

[d] LEV and PYR have only a limited effect on trichuriasis but, when used in combination with oxantel, PYR has an efficacy against trichuriasis comparable to that observed with MBD (14).

3.2 Ancillary benefits and advantages of preventive chemotherapy

Preventive chemotherapy targeted at lymphatic filariasis, onchocerciasis, schistosomiasis and soil-transmitted helminthiasis not only reduces the morbidity caused by those diseases but also yields a number of ancillary benefits and advantages, outlined below.

- Relief from other helminth infections, and from ectoparasitic infections such as scabies and lice, will follow, with commensurate health benefits (see Table 1).
- Community compliance within other health-care programmes will be increased and school attendance improved (*15–17*).
- Epidemiological evidence strongly suggests that
  - the establishment of HIV infection and acceleration to AIDS will be reduced when schistosomiasis and soil-transmitted helminth infections are treated (*11, 12, 18*);
  - treatment of soil-transmitted helminth infections will help to lessen the burden of malaria (*10, 19*);
  - treatment of helminth infections may help to lessen the burden of tuberculosis (*11*).

Sustained, large-scale preventive chemotherapy against helminthic infections is a cost-effective intervention that contributes to the achievement of several Millennium Development Goals (*20, 21*) including:

1. eradicating extreme poverty and hunger
2. achieving universal primary education
3. promoting gender equality
4. reducing child mortality
5. improving maternal health and
6. combating HIV/AIDS, malaria and tuberculosis.

References

1. *Report of the Fifth Meeting of the Technical Advisory Group on the Global Elimination of Lymphatic Filariasis.* Geneva, World Health Organization, 2004 (CDS/CPE/CEE/2004.42).

2. Cook GC, Zumla AI, eds. *Manson's tropical diseases*, 21st ed. London, Saunders, 2003.

3. Perel Y et al. Utilisation des collecteurs urinaires chez les enfants de 0 à 4 ans en enquête de masse sur la schistosomose urinaire au Niger [Use of urine collectors for infants from 0 to 4 years of age in a mass survey of urinary schistosomiasis in Niger]. *Médecine Tropicale*, 1985, 45:429–433.

4. Bosompem KM et al. Infant schistosomiasis in Ghana: a survey in an irrigation community. *Tropical Medicine and International Health*, 2004, 9:917–922.

5. Odogwu SE et al. Intestinal schistosomiasis in infants (<3 years of age) along the Ugandan shoreline of Lake Victoria. *Annals of Tropical Medicine and Parasitology*, 2006, 100: 315–326.

6. Witt C, Ottesen EA. Lymphatic filariasis: an infection of childhood. *Tropical Medicine and International Health*, 2001, 6:582–606.

7. Albonico M, Crompton DW, Savioli L. Control strategies for human intestinal nematode infections. *Advances in Parasitology*, 1999, 42:277–341.

8. King CH, Dickman K, Tisch DJ. Reassessment of the cost of chronic helminthic infection: a meta-analysis of disability-related outcomes in endemic schistosomiasis. *Lancet*, 2005, 365:1561–1569.

9. Hotez PJ et al. Helminth infections: soil-transmitted helminth infections and schistosomiasis. In: *Disease control priorities in developing countries*, 2nd ed. Oxford, Oxford University Press, 2006. Available at http://www.dcp2.org accessed 18 August 2006.

10. Druilhe P, Tall A, Sokhna C. Worms can worsen malaria: towards a new means to roll back malaria? *Trends in Parasitology*, 2005, 21:359–362.

11. Fincham JE, Markus MB, Adams VJ. Could control of soil-transmitted helminthic infection influence the HIV/AIDS pandemic? *Acta Tropica*, 2003, 86:315–333.

12. Kjetland EF et al. Association between genital schistosomiasis and HIV in rural Zimbabwean women. *AIDS*, 2006, 20:593–600.

13. Mehta DK, Ryan RSM, Hogerzeil HV, eds. *WHO Model Formulary 2004*. Geneva, World Health Organization, 2004.

14. Albonico M et al. Evaluation of the efficacy of pyrantel-oxantel for the treatment of soil-transmitted nematode infections. *Transactions of the Royal Society of Tropical Medicine and Hygiene*, 2002, 96:685–690.

15. de Clercq D et al. The relationship between *Schistosoma haematobium* infection and school performance and attendance in Bamako, Mali. *Annals of Tropical Medicine and Parasitology*, 1998, 92:851–858.

16. Jancloes M. The case for control: forging a partnership with decision-makers. In: Crompton DWT, Nesheim MC, Pawlowski ZS, eds. *Ascariasis and its prevention and control*. London, Taylor & Francis, 1989.

17. Sakti H et al. Evidence for an association between hookworm infection and cognitive function in Indonesian school children. *Tropical Medicine and International Health*, 1999, 4:322–334.

18. Kallestrup P et al. Schistosomiasis and HIV-1 infection in rural Zimbabwe: effect of treatment of schistosomiasis on CD4 cell count and plasma HIV-1 RNA load. *Journal of Infectious Diseases*, 2005, 192:1956–1961.

19. Spiegel A et al. Increased frequency of malaria attacks in subjects co-infected by intestinal worms and *Plasmodium falciparum* malaria. *Transactions of the Royal Society of Tropical Medicine and Hygiene*, 2003, 97:198–199.

20. *United Nations Millennium Declaration*. New York, NY, United Nations, 2000 (A/RES/55/2; http://www.un-ngls.org/MDG/A-RES-55-2.pdf, accessed 18 August 2006).

21. *Report of the third global meeting of the partners for parasite control. Deworming for health and development*. Geneva, World Health Organization, 2005 (WHO/CDS/CPE/PVC/2005.14).

4. WHO-RECOMMENDED DRUGS: ALONE AND IN COMBINATION

A selection of anthelminthic drugs is available for use in public health programmes designed to control helminth infections and reduce morbidity (Table 1). Several of these drugs have been made available through the generosity of a number of pharmaceutical companies. Other drugs are available as good-quality, low-cost generic products, now that patent protection has expired. For example, a tablet of generic albendazole (400 mg) or mebendazole (500 mg) costs as little as US$ 0.02. Information on WHO-recommended drugs, dosages, implementation thresholds and regimens in preventive chemotherapy is summarized in Table 2.

Table 2. **Drugs, dosages, implementation thresholds and regimens in preventive chemotherapy interventions**

Note: Drug names are given in full in the list of abbreviations at the front of the manual.

Disease	Drugs and dosages	Threshold for implementation of preventive chemotherapy interventions[b]	Frequency of intervention
Lymphatic filariasis (in countries where onchocerciasis is co-endemic)	IVM according to height (using IVM tablet-pole) **plus** ALB 400 mg	Prevalence of infection ≥1%	Once a year
Lymphatic filariasis (in countries where onchocerciasis is not co-endemic)	DEC 6 mg/kg (using age as criterion for dose) **plus** ALB 400 mg	Prevalence of infection ≥1%	Once a year
Onchocerciasis	IVM according to height (using IVM tablet-pole)	Prevalence of infection ≥ 40% or prevalence of palpable nodules ≥ 20%	Once a year
Schistosomiasis	PZQ 40 mg/kg (using PZQ tablet-pole)	Presence of infection	According to prevalence of infection (see Annex 2)
Soil-transmitted helminthiasis (ascariasis, trichuriasis, hookworm disease)	ALB 400 mg **or** MBD 500 mg[a]	Prevalence of infection ≥ 20%	According to prevalence of infection (see Annex 2)
Trachoma	Azilthromycin 20mg/kg (using tablet-pole) max 1g in adults	Active trachoma (TF) prevalence > 5 % in 1–9 years old at district level[c]	Once a year

[a] LEV 2.5 mg/kg or PYR 10 mg/kg is useful where trichuriasis does not pose a significant problem.
[b] For details, see Annex 6.
[c] TF >10% at district level: dictrict-wide mass treatment. If TF <5% at district level, some communities might still require community wide treatment.

5. PREVENTIVE CHEMOTHERAPY: BEST PRACTICE

5.1 Eligibility and ineligibility for treatment

Information and details on eligible and ineligible populations for large-scale preventive chemotherapy interventions are provided on pages 20–26.

5.2 Safety and adverse reactions

Millions of doses of anthelminthics have been used since registration of these drugs for human treatment was approved (*1*). Each drug has an excellent safety record; adverse reactions are minimal and transient, and serious adverse experiences are extremely infrequent. In practice, both infected and uninfected people are treated in community programmes. Temporary minor reactions following treatment occur mainly in infected people and usually result from the body's response to the dying of worms: heavily infected people are more likely to experience such reactions (*2*, *3*). Generally, the number of people reporting adverse reactions is highest at the first round of treatment and tends to decrease during subsequent rounds (*4*).

The following general precautionary measures are recommended to ensure the smooth and safe implementation of large-scale drug delivery programmes:

■ Seriously ill individuals (people unable to engage in the normal activities of daily living without assistance because of their illnesses) should be excluded from large-scale anthelminthic treatment interventions.

■ Programme managers must ensure that people who are about to receive drugs are adequately informed about possible adverse reactions and about what they should do in the event of such a reaction.

■ People who have previously suffered one of the rare serious adverse experiences caused by reaction to the drugs (e.g. Stevens–Johnson syndrome) should be excluded from treatment.

■ Programme managers must ensure that care and support are available for individuals who experience adverse reactions. It is important that medical or community health personnel are available throughout the rounds of treatment.

■ Any serious adverse experience should be carefully recorded and the relevant authorities should be informed. An example of a recording form for serious adverse experiences is provided in Annex 3.

■ Scored tablets should be broken into smaller pieces, or crushed, for administration to young children; older children should be encouraged to chew tablets of albendazole or mebendazole. Forcing very small children to swallow large tablets may cause choking or asphyxiation.

■ Programme managers should be aware of any other public health intervention that is distributing drugs in the same area and of its timing. This is to minimize the risk of targeted people suffering from adverse reactions due to interactions between drugs distributed by different programmes.

5.2.1 Safety of drug combinations for treatment of helminth infections

A number of studies have investigated the safety of drug combinations in the treatment of helminth infections:

- Albendazole and praziquantel can be safely co-administered for schistosomiasis and soil-transmitted helminthiasis (5).
- Mebendazole and praziquantel have been widely co-administered in many countries and reported to be safe (6–8).
- Albendazole plus ivermectin can be safely used for the treatment of lymphatic filariasis (9–12).
- Albendazole plus diethylcarbamazine (DEC) is also a safe combination in the treatment of lymphatic filariasis (10, 13, 14).

Preliminary assessments of the co-administration of the three drugs (albendazole, ivermectin and praziquantel) indicate that there is no clinically relevant pharmacokinetic interaction between the three drugs when given concurrently as single oral doses in healthy volunteers; no additional adverse reactions are therefore expected as a result of their co-administration in non-infected individuals (15). However, some precautionary measures should be observed when infected populations are co-administred with the three-or the two-drug combination (see Box B).

For the use of albendazole plus ivermectin in *Loa loa* endemic areas, please see section 5.6.

Box B. Co-administration of albendazole, ivermectin and praziquantel

In some instances, co-administration of albendazole, ivermectin and praziquantel would provide evident operational advantages. However, the following precautions should be exercised:

- In a population that has never been subjected to mass treatment with any of these drugs, the initial 1–2 rounds of treatment with praziquantel should be given separately from albendazole and/or ivermectin treatment;[a]
- In a population that has previously been subjected to (separate) mass treatment with praziquantel and ivermectin or praziquantel and ivermectin+albendazole, extra safety monitoring should be carried out during the initial rounds of large-scale combined treatment to monitor for any unanticipated adverse reactions.

The same precautions should be taken in case of co-admistration of ivermectin and praziquantel.

[a] Co-administration of PZQ and ALB (in SCH and STH control) and of IVM and ALB (in LF elimination) has already been approved for all circumstances.

5.2.2 Safety in pregnancy

Several studies have failed to find a statistically significant difference in the occurrence of congenital abnormalities between babies born to women treated with single-dose mebendazole or albendazole during pregnancy and those born to untreated women (*16–20*). Similarly, no significant difference has been found in the occurrence of adverse birth outcomes (abortion, stillbirth, birth defects) between women inadvertently exposed to praziquantel, ivermectin, or the combination of ivermectin and albendazole (during large-scale chemotherapy interventions), and women not exposed to the drugs (*21–24*). These studies include approximately 6000 documented exposures to mebendazole, but the number of documented exposures to the other anthelminthic drugs is much lower (approximately 50–200). Very little is currently known about the effects of DEC, levamisole and pyrantel on birth outcome, but 50 years' experience of treating hundreds of millions of people with DEC suggests the safety of this drug in women inadvertently exposed to it during pregnancy. For current recommendations on the use of anthelminthic drugs in pregnancy, see section 5.5.3.

5.3 Drug quality

Programme managers must procure good-quality drugs according to the recommended pharmacopoeia from manufacturers who practise certified good manufacturing practice (GMP) and good laboratory practice (GLP). Wherever possible, drugs should be procured from prequalified suppliers. Ministries of health can seek assistance from WHO's procurement services, if no such local manufacturers are available. All procurements by WHO or UNICEF, for both donated and purchased drugs, apply these standard practices. When drugs are acquired from less established sources or through occasional small-scale donations, guarantees of quality should be sought (*25, 26*).

5.4 Programme implementation

5.4.1 Drug delivery and incorporation into established and novel programmes

Drug delivery involves:
1. calculating the number of doses required for each round of treatment, with provision for loss and wastage;
2. establishing a mechanism for distributing the drugs to the agreed collection points on the due date; and
3. mobilizing active community participation in the entire process.

A secure system must be in place for storage of drugs under conditions that prevent deterioration. An inventory of drug supplies, batch numbers, and expiry dates should be maintained for stock rotation to minimize the quantity of stocks reaching its expiry date. One person – or preferably two people – must be designated to keep accurate records of drug consignments during rounds of treatment. Information about sources of drug supply is given in Annex 4.

A reliable and sustainable mechanism must be agreed for moving consignments of drugs from their place of manufacture, through the national port of entry, to the communities identified for treatment. Funds must be available to cover costs at the time of drug arrival in the country. Whenever possible, distribution should take advantage of the national delivery system and existing community organizations. The costs of this logistic phase of a programme must not be ignored. Most drug donations are exempt from import duty and other taxes. Every effort should therefore be made to establish such an arrangement if it is not already in place; otherwise, provision must be made for paying the taxes or levies.

Preventive chemotherapy interventions will be more effective, and compliance with subsequent rounds of treatment sustained, if communities are properly informed about the aims and objectives of the programme. The results of knowledge, attitudes and practices – or KAP – surveys can provide programme managers with information about health awareness among people in need of treatment. Communities also need to be aware of the purpose of drug administration, the timing and location of treatment rounds, and the measures to be taken if any adverse events should occur. Clear and concise messages to the community about preventive chemotherapy programmes should be delivered in a socially appropriate manner and in time to reach as many people as possible.

In many places, there may be opportunities to associate preventive chemotherapy interventions with existing health-care programmes that make use of different drug distribution channels. Campaigns targeting mothers and children, such as those distributing vitamin A and insecticide-treated nets, vaccination outreach services, child or mother-and-child health days, antenatal clinics and school health programmes, may offer an inexpensive approach for regular anthelminthic drug administration (*27, 28*). In most instances, interventions that are "packaged" in this way yield additional benefits (*29–31*).

It may also be possible to associate trachoma control programmes where these exist – *with the caution* that the safety of large-scale co-administration of azithromycin and anthelminthic drugs cannot be guaranteed by current knowledge and is being further investigated. The available information indicates that a sufficient clearing time must be respected when azithromycin and anthelminthic drugs are administered to the same population.

Community-wide drug distribution programmes that use existing health systems, community-based approaches, or both – such as those for lymphatic filariasis and onchocerciasis – may also offer opportunities to expand preventive chemotherapy interventions by including distribution of other anthelminthic drugs.

In reality, the numbers of trained health personnel available may be insufficient to carry out drug administration to the many people in need of preventive chemotherapy. The safety record of anthelminthic drugs and ease of administration allow this obstacle to be overcome by elementary training of non-medically qualified people such as schoolteachers, traditional healers and community volunteers (*32, 33*). Programme managers, in consultation with target communities, should develop the method of drug delivery and administration that is best suited to local conditions.

5.4.2   Implementation charts – how to intervene

Following the assessment of the helminthiasis burden, a coordinated plan of action for intervention should be prepared at the district and community levels using the following charts (algorithms and boxes) as a reference. The algorithms suggest the possible epidemiological combinations of the four helminthic diseases, and the necessary action, in areas where lymphatic filariasis is endemic (Algorithm 1) and in areas where lymphatic filariasis is not endemic (Algorithm 2). The subsequent boxes show the details of each intervention recommended by the relevant algorithm (MDA1, MDA2, MDA3, T1, T2, T3).

The evidence used as the basis for each recommendation is summarized below each box. The symbols used (in order of level of evidence) are as follows:

S   formal systematic reviews, such as a Cochrane review, including more than one randomized controlled trial;

T   comparative trials without formal systematic review;

O   observational studies (e.g. surveillance or pharmacological data);

E   expert opinion/consensus.

Algorithm 1 – Coordinated implementation of preventive chemotherapy interventions

LF +

ONCHO +

SCH +

STH high   STH low   STH −

MDA1 T1	MDA1 T2	MDA1 T2

SCH −

STH high   STH low   STH −

MDA1 T3	MDA1	MDA1

ONCHO −

SCH +

STH high   STH low   STH −

MDA1/2ᵃT1	MDA1/2ᵃ T2	MDA1/2ᵃ T2

SCH −

STH high   STH low   STH −

MDA1/2ᵃT3	MDA1/2ᵃ	MDA1/2ᵃ

Legend

Mass drug administration

MDA1ᵃ   IVM+ALB
MDA2ᵃ   DEC+ALB
MDA3   IVM

Targeted treatment

T1   ALB+PZQ or MBD+PZQ
T2   PZQ
T3   ALB or MBD

Colour coding

Yellow: first annual drug distribution
Green: second annual drug distribution, to be carried out 6 months after the first annual drug distribution
Blue: second annual drug distribution, to be carried out anytime, but at least 1 week after the first annual drug distribution. In some instances ALB, IVM and PZQ can be coadministred. See Box B, page 14.

ᵃ MDA1/2: if the country is endemic for ONCHO, IVM (instead of DEC) should be used to control LF even if ONCHO is not transmitted in the targeted areas. To control LF, therefore, IVM should be used in ONCHO-endemic countries (MDA1) and DEC in ONCHO-free countries (MDA2), irrespective of whether ONCHO is transmitted in the targeted area.

Algorithm 2 – Coordinated implementation of preventive chemotherapy interventions

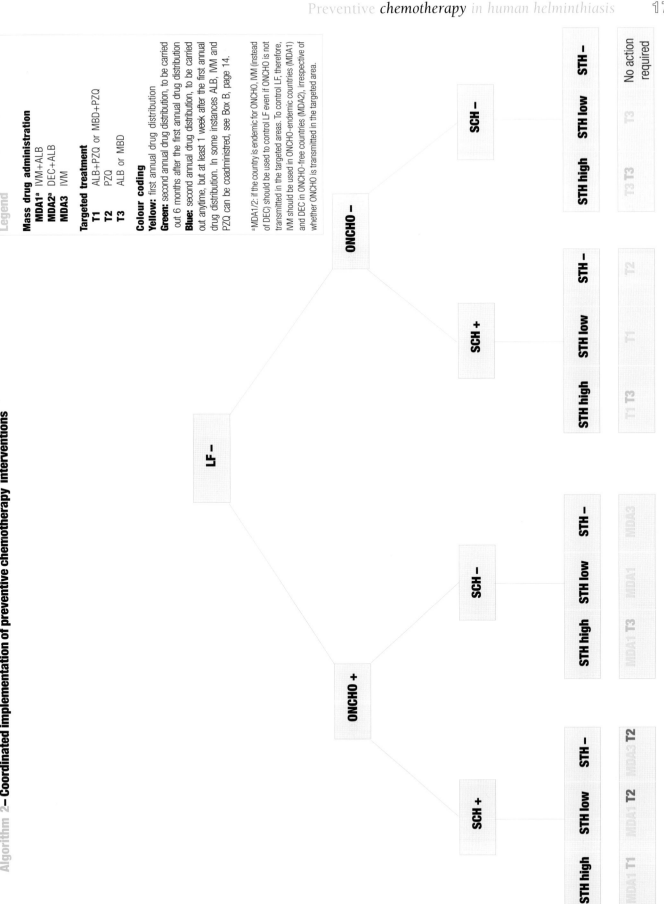

Legend

Mass drug administration
MDA1[a] IVM+ALB
MDA2[a] DEC+ALB
MDA3 IVM

Targeted treatment
T1 ALB+PZQ or MBD+PZQ
T2 PZQ
T3 ALB or MBD

Colour coding
Yellow: first annual drug distribution
Green: second annual drug distribution, to be carried out 6 months after the first annual drug distribution
Blue: second annual drug distribution, to be carried out anytime, but at least 1 week after the first annual drug distribution. In some instances ALB, IVM and PZQ can be coadministred, see Box B, page 14.

[a] MDA1/2: if the country is endemic for ONCHO, IVM (instead of DEC) should be used to control LF even if ONCHO is not transmitted in the targeted areas. To control LF, therefore, IVM should be used in ONCHO-endemic countries (MDA1) and DEC in ONCHO-free countries (MDA2), irrespective of whether ONCHO is transmitted in the targeted area.

Intervention MDA1

Diseases targeted

lymphatic filariasis or
lymphatic filariasis and onchocerciasis or
lymphatic filariasis and soil-transmitted helminthiasis or
lymphatic filariasis and onchocerciasis and soil-transmitted helminthiasis

Drug(s)

ivermectin and albendazole, administered together

Frequency of implementation

Repeated at yearly intervals.

Eligible population

The entire population at risk of LF transmission, i.e. the entire population in an area where LF transmission occurs (implementation unit), except those excluded (see ineligible population).

Ineligible population

Pregnant women, lactating women in the first week after birth, children <90 cm in height (approximately equivalent to a weight of 15 kg), and the severely ill.

Co-administration of IVM and ALB in areas where *Loa loa* is endemic[a]

In areas where *Loa loa* is endemic, caution is essential in the use of IVM because of the risk of encephalopathy in individuals with high levels Loa microfilaraemia. The following measures are therefore recommended:

■ Potential *Loa* endemicity in the area targeted for IVM treatment should be assessed using the RAPLOA[b] methodology. (Countries where *Loa loa* has been reported are listed in Annex 1).

■ *Where RAPLOA is positive but under 40% (i.e. prevalence of eye worm history is <40%)*, the communities targeted for MDA with IVM (those where ONCHO is meso- and hyperendemic) should be made aware of, and educated about, the possibility of serious adverse experiences (SAEs); personnel involved should be trained in the recognition, reporting, referral and general management of SAE cases (*passive surveillance*).

■ *Where RAPLOA is 40% or more (i.e. prevalence of eye worm history is ≥40%)*, the above recommendations also apply: in addition, referral hospitals for SAE management should be designated and properly equipped and should have trained medical staff (*enhanced passive surveillance*).

■ In areas where ONCHO is hypo-endemic and there is no MDA, clinic-based IVM treatment can be given provided that each patient is individually assessed for ONCHO and loiasis, is properly informed about possible SAEs, and is kept under surveillance.

■ There is no biological rationale or available data to suggest that addition of ALB to MDA interventions with IVM in areas where *Loa loa* is endemic would increase the number or severity of SAEs if the two drugs were used together to treat populations in areas co-endemic for ONCHO, LF and loiasis. However, the following additional surveillance measures are recommended when the IVM+ALB combination is used in loiasis-endemic areas:

• *In areas where two or more MDAs have already been carried out with IVM alone with good coverage,*[1] levels of *Loa loa* microfilaraemia are likely to be far below those associated with encephalopathy and other SAEs. It can be recommended that the addition of ALB could proceed with <u>enhanced passive surveillance</u>, as currently recommended for IVM administration for ONCHO in *Loa*-endemic areas where RAPLOA is ≥40%.

• *In areas where there has been no previous MDA with IVM alone, where there has been one MDA with IVM alone, or where previous coverage has been poor*, there should be <u>active surveillance</u>, similar to that at the start of the global LF elimination programme, until at least 15 000 individuals have been assessed.[2]

[a] For further information, see: Mectizan® Expert Committee/Technical Consultative Committee. Recommendations for the treatment of onchocerciasis with Mectizan® in areas co-endemic for onchocerciasis and loiasis, June 2004. Decatur, GA, Mectizan® Expert Committee/ Mectizan® Donation Program, 2004 (available at http://www.mectizan.org/library/EnglishMECTCCLoaRecs-June04.pdf; accessed July 2006) and Mectizan® Expert Committee/Albendazole Coordination. *Report of 35th Meeting, London, United Kingdom, January 10–12, 2006.*

[b] For further information on RAPLOA, see: *Guidelines for rapid assessment of Loa loa.* Geneva, World Health Organization, 2002 (TDR/IDE/RAPLOA/02.1).

[1] Defined as 65% therapeutic coverage of total population or 80% therapeutic coverage of the eligible population.
[2] This active surveillance initiative should be undertaken only in areas where all the medical safety mechanisms for handling potential SAEs are well established.

Levels of evidence

- **Lymphatic filariasis**
  S: *13, 14, 24, 34–40*
- **Onchocerciasis**
  S: *41, 42, 46*
  T: *43–45*
  O: *47–49*
  E: *50, 51*
- **Soil-transmitted helminthiasis**
  S: *52*
  E: *53*

Intervention MDA2

Diseases targeted
lymphatic filariasis or
lymphatic filariasis and soil-transmitted helminthiasis
Drug(s)
diethylcarbamazine and albendazole, administered together
Frequency of implementation
Repeated at yearly intervals.
Eligible population
The entire population at risk of LF transmission, i.e. the entire population in an area where LF transmission occurs
(implementation unit), except those excluded (see ineligible population).
Ineligible population
Pregnant women, children under 2 years of age, and the severely ill.

Levels of evidence

- **Lymphatic filariasis**
  S: *13, 14, 24, 34–40*
- **Soil-transmitted helminthiasis**
  S: *52*
  E: *53*

Intervention MDA3

Diseases targeted
> onchocerciasis

Drug(s)
> ivermectin

Frequency of implementation
> Repeated at yearly intervals (standard option); in some countries, the national plan recommends administration of IVM at 6-monthly intervals.

Eligible population
> The entire population in meso-and hyperendemic communities (prevalence of infection ≥40% or prevalence of palpable nodules ≥20%), except those excluded (see ineligible population).

Ineligible population
> Pregnant women, lactating women in the first week after birth, children <90 cm in height (approximately equivalent to a weight of 15 kg), and the severely ill.

Use of IVM in areas where *Loa loa* is endemic[a]

In areas where *Loa loa* is endemic, caution is essential in the use of IVM because of the risk of encephalopathy in individuals with high levels of *Loa* microfilaraemia. The following measures are therefore recommended:

■ Potential *Loa* endemicity in the area targeted for IVM treatment should be assessed using the RAPLOA[b] methodology. (Countries where *Loa loa* has been reported are listed in Annex 1).

■ *Where RAPLOA is positive but under 40% (i.e. prevalence of eye worm history is <40%)*, the communities targeted for MDA with IVM (those where ONCHO is meso- and hyperendemic) should be made aware of, and educated about, the possibility of severe adverse experiences (SAEs); personnel involved should be trained in the recognition, reporting, referral and general management of SAE cases (*passive surveillance*).

■ *Where RAPLOA is 40% or more (i.e. the prevalence of eye worm history is ≥40%)*, the above recommendations also apply; in addition, referral hospitals for SAE management should be designated and properly equipped and should have trained medical staff (*enhanced passive surveillance*).

■ In areas where ONCHO is hypo-endemic and there is no MDA, clinic-based IVM treatment can be given provided that each patient is individually assessed for ONCHO and loiasis, is properly informed about possible SAEs, and is kept under surveillance.

[a] For further information, see: Mectizan® Expert Committee/Technical Consultative Committee. *Recommendations for the treatment of onchocerciasis with Mectizan® in areas co-endemic for onchocerciasis and loiasis, June 2004*. Decatur, GA, Mectizan® Expert Committee/ Mectizan® Donation Program, 2004. (available at http://www.mectizan.org/library/EnglishMECTCCLoaRecs-June04.pdf; accessed July 2006).
[b] For further information on RAPLOA, see: *Guidelines for rapid assessment of Loa loa*. Geneva, World Health Organization, 2002 (TDR/IDE/RAPLOA/02.1).

Levels of evidence

- **Onchocerciasis**

  S: *41, 42, 46*

  T: *43–45*

  O: *47–49*

  E: *50, 51*

Intervention T1

Diseases targeted

schistosomiasis and soil-transmitted helminthiasis

Drug(s)

praziquantel **and** albendazole or mebendazole, administered together

Frequency of implementation

Once or twice a year for ALB or MBD. The frequency of PZQ varies according to the risk of SCH: PZQ treatment should take place once a year in high-risk communities, once every 2 years in moderate-risk communities, and twice during the period of primary schooling age in low-risk communities.

Eligible population for PZQ

- School-age children.
- Adults considered to be at risk, from special groups (pregnant and lactating women; groups with occupations involving contact with infested water, such as fishermen, farmers, irrigation workers, or women in their domestic tasks) to entire communities living in endemic areas.

Ineligible population for PZQ

There is no documented information on the safety of PZQ for children under 4 years of age (or under 94 cm in height). These children should therefore be excluded from mass treatment but can be treated on an individual basis by medical personnel.

Eligible population for ALB or MBD

Preschool and school-age children; women of childbearing age (including pregnant women in the 2nd and 3rd trimesters and lactating women); adults at high risk in certain occupations (e.g. tea-pickers and miners).

Ineligible population for ALB or MBD

Children in the 1st year of life; pregnant women in the 1st trimester of pregnancy.

Note 1: If a second annual T1 campaign is to be carried out, it should take place 6 months after the first. In communities at very high risk, a third annual campaign distributing ALB or MBD (T3) may be added. In this case the appropriate frequency of the three annual campaigns would be every 4 months.

Note 2: Levamisole or pyrantel may also be used instead of ALB or MBD.

Levels of evidence

- **Schistosomiasis and soil-transmitted helminthiasis**

    S: *52*

    O: *6, 7*

    E: *53*

Intervention T2

Diseases targeted
schistosomiasis

Drug(s)
praziquantel

Frequency of implementation
Varies according to the risk of SCH: T2 should take place once a year in high-risk communities, once every 2 years in moderate-risk communities, and twice during the period of primary schooling age in low-risk communities.

Eligible population
School-age children.

Adults considered to be at risk, from special groups (pregnant and lactating women; groups with occupations involving contact with infested water, such as fishermen, farmers, irrigation workers, or women in their domestic tasks) to entire communities living in endemic areas.

Ineligible population
There is no documented information on the safety of PZQ for children under 4 years of age (or under 94 cm in height). These children should therefore be excluded from mass treatment but can be treated on an individual basis by medical personnel.

Note : T2 as second annual campaign can take place at any time, but at least 1 week after the first annual campaign. There may be opportunities to add PZQ treatment to MDA1 in certain circumstances (see Box B).

Levels of evidence

- **Schistosomiasis**
    S: *52*
    O: *6, 7*
    E: *53*

Intervention T3

Diseases targeted
>soil-transmitted helminthiasis

Drug(s)
>albendazole or mebendazole

Frequency of implementation
>Once or twice per year (see algorithms 1 and 2).

Eligible population
>Preschool and school-age children; women of childbearing age (including pregnant women in the 2nd and 3rd trimesters and lactating women); adults at high risk in certain occupations (e.g. tea-pickers and miners).

Ineligible population
>Children in the 1st year of life; pregnant women in the 1st trimester of pregnancy.

Note 1: If a second annual T3 campaign is to be carried out, it should take place 6 months after the first. In communities at very high risk, a third annual campaign distributing ALB or MBD may be added. In this case the appropriate frequency of the three annual campaigns would be every 4 months.

Note 2: Levamisole or pyrantel may also be used instead of albendazole or mebendazole.

Levels of evidence

- **Soil-transmitted helminthiasis**

  S: *52*

  E: *53*

The following sections offer guidance on preventive chemotherapy for different age groups and special risk groups. The dosages apply to large-scale treatment programmes without diagnosis (see also Table A4.1).

5.5.1   Preschool children (aged 1–5 years)

ALB   200 mg for children aged 12–23 months (*54, 55*)
       400 mg for children aged 2–5 years (*54, 55*)

MBD   500 mg for children aged ≥1 year (*54, 55*)

LEV   2.5 mg/kg for children aged ≥1 year (*54, 55*)

PYR   10 mg/kg for children aged ≥1 year (*54, 55*)

PZQ   according to height for children aged ≥4 years or ≥94 cm (refer to PZQ dose pole, designed to deliver a dose of at least 40mg/kg) (*56, 57*)

IVM   according to height for children ≥15 kg or ≥90 cm (refer to IVM dose pole) (*32, 58*)

DEC[1] 6mg/kg for children aged ≥2 years (*55*)
       standard dose for children aged 2 to 5 years 100 mg (*59*)

5.5.2   School-age children (aged 6–15 years) and adults (aged >15 years)

ALB   400 mg (*55*)

MBD   500 mg (*55*)

LEV   2.5 mg/kg
       standard dose for school-age children 80 mg (*33, 55*)

PYR   10 mg/kg (*55*)

PZQ   according to height starting from ≥94 cm (refer to PZQ dose pole) (*56, 57*)

IVM   according to height starting from a weight ≥15 kg or a height ≥90 cm (refer to IVM dose pole) (*32, 58*)

DEC[1] 6mg/kg (*55*)
       standard dose for school-age children 200 mg (*59*)
       standard dose for adults 300 mg (*59*)

---

[1] These doses are intended only as a guide, since health authorities in many countries have developed their own specific treatment regimens.

5.5.3 Adolescent girls, women of reproductive age and pregnant women

Despite excellent empirical safety profiles, none of the anthelminthic drugs considered in this manual is licensed for use in pregnancy or in the first trimester of pregnancy; thus there remains ambiguity about the ethics of exposing women of reproductive age to such drugs. Women have the right to refuse or delay treatment if they are unsure about pregnancy, and programmes must ensure that treatment is subsequently available to women who choose to exercise this right.

In areas where schistosomiasis and soil-transmitted helminthiasis are endemic, risk–benefit analyses have revealed that the health advantages of treating women of reproductive age and pregnant women far outweigh the risks to their health and to the health of their babies (*60*). The benefits of treating pregnant women include reduced maternal anaemia (*19, 20*) and improved infant birth weight and survival (*61*). The proven benefits of antenatal deworming in the absence of any evidence indicative of drug teratogenicity or embryotoxicity in humans (see section 5.2.2 for details) provides compelling evidence to support the treatment with albendazole or mebendazole of women for STH after the first trimester of pregnancy (*16–20, 60–63*). Evidence also shows that women can be treated with praziquantel at any stage of pregnancy and during lactation (*5, 54, 64, 65*).

The exclusion of drug combinations involving either DEC or ivermectin in relation to pregnancy is a necessary precaution in the absence of definitive safety information. This manual recommends that programme managers consider pregnant women as ineligible for treatment with the drug combinations IVM+ALB or DEC+ALB or with IVM alone, in preventive chemotherapy interventions against lymphatic filariasis and/or onchocerciasis. IVM+ALB or IVM alone should also not be given to lactating women in the first week after birth.

Programme managers are, however, encouraged to include pregnant women at any stage of pregnancy and during lactation in preventive chemotherapy interventions distributing praziquantel against schistosomiasis.

For soil-transmitted helminthiasis, this manual recommends that albendazole or mebendazole be offered to pregnant women in the 2nd and 3rd trimesters of pregnancy and to lactating women in preventive chemotherapy interventions targeting areas where the prevalence of any soil-transmitted helminth infection (ascariasis, trichuriasis and hookworm infection) exceeds 20%.

Every effort must be made to avoid excluding from treatment eligible adolescents and women of reproductive age. For identification of women who are pregnant and for definition of the stage of pregnancy, the date of a woman's last menstrual period has proved reliable (*66, 67*).

5.6   Problems caused by concurrent infections

Programme managers should be aware that sustainable anthelminthic treatment for lymphatic filariasis, onchocerciasis, schistosomiasis and soil-transmitted helminthiasis may be disrupted if serious adverse experiences occur as a result of the inadvertent treatment of certain concurrent infections that have not been recognized (e.g. following praziquantel treatment of neurocysticercosis). The following precautionary measures are therefore recommended:

PZQ

As praziquantel can exacerbate central nervous system pathology due to schistosomiasis, paragonimiasis or *Taenia solium* cysticercosis, as a general rule this drug should not be administered in large-scale interventions to individuals reporting a history of epilepsy and/or other signs of potential central nervous system involvement such as subcutaneous nodules suggestive of cystercosis (*55*).

IVM in loiasis-endemic areas

Special measures should be taken when ivermectin alone is used in MDA interventions against onchocerciasis in areas where *Loa loa* is endemic (*68*). See intervention MDA3 box in section 5.4.2 for further details.

IVM+ALB in loiasis-endemic areas

The same special measures should also be taken when ivermectin is used in combination with albendazole in MDA interventions against lymphatic filariasis and onchocerciasis in areas where *Loa loa* is endemic. There is no biological rationale or available data to suggest that the addition of albendazole to MDA interventions with ivermectin in areas where *Loa loa* is endemic would increase the number or severity of SAEs if the two drugs were to be used together to treat populations co-endemic for onchocerciasis, lymphatic filariasis and loiasis. However, special surveillance measures are recommended (*69*). See intervention MDA1 box in section 5.4.2 for further details.

References

1. Stephenson LS et al., eds. Controlling intestinal helminths while eliminating lymphatic filariasis. *Parasitology*, 2000, 121(Suppl.):S1–S173.

2. Report on active surveillance for adverse events following the use of drug co-administrations in the Global Programme to Eliminate Lymphatic Filariasis. *Weekly Epidemiological Record*, 2003, 78:315–317.

3. Loukas A, Hotez PJ. Chemotherapy of helminth infections. In: Brunton LL et al., eds. *Goodman and Gilman's The pharmacological basis of therapeutics*, 11th ed. New York, McGraw-Hill, 2006.

4. Beau de Rochars M et al. The Leogane, Haiti, demonstration project: decreased microfilaremia and program costs after three years of mass drug administration. *American Journal of Tropical Medicine and Hygiene*, 2005, 73:888–894.

5. Olds GR. Administration of praziquantel to pregnant and lactating women. *Acta Tropica*, 2003, 86:185–195.

6. Engels D, Ndoricimpa J, Gryseels B. Schistosomiasis mansoni in Burundi: progress in its control since 1985. *Bulletin of the World Health Organization*, 1993, 71:207–214.

7. Engels D et al. Control of *Schistosoma mansoni* and intestinal helminths: 8-year follow-up of an urban school programme in Bujumbura, Burundi. *Acta Tropica*, 1994, 58:127–140.

8. *The Partnership for Parasite Control. Notes of the Second Meeting, Rome*, 25–26 April 2002. Geneva, World Health Organization, 2002.

9. Awadzi K et al. The co-administration of ivermectin and albendazole – safety, pharmacokinetics and efficacy against *Onchocerca volvulus*. *Annals of Tropical Medicine and Parasitology*, 2003, 97:165–178.

10. Horton J et al. An analysis of the safety of the single dose, two drug regimens used in programmes to eliminate lymphatic filariasis. In: Stephenson LS et al., eds. Controlling intestinal helminths while eliminating lymphatic filariasis. *Parasitology*, 2000, 121(Suppl.):S147–S160.

11. Kshirsagar NA et al. Safety, tolerability, efficacy and plasma concentrations of diethylcarbamazine and albendazole co-administration in a field study in an area endemic for lymphatic filariasis in India. *Transactions of the Royal Society of Tropical Medicine and Hygiene*, 2004, 98:205–217.

12. Simonsen PE et al. The effect of single dose ivermectin alone or in combination with albendazole on *Wuchereria bancrofti* infection in primary school children in Tanzania. *Transactions of the Royal Society of Tropical Medicine and Hygiene*, 2004, 98:462–472.

13. *Report of the Third Meeting of the Technical Advisory Group on the Global Elimination of Lymphatic Filariasis*. Geneva, World Health Organization, 2002.

14. *Report of the Fourth Meeting of the Technical Advisory Group on the Global Elimination of Lymphatic Filariasis*. Geneva, World Health Organization, 2003 (CDS/CPE/CEE/2003.39).

15. Na-Bangchang K et al. Assessment of pharmacokinetic drug interactions and tolerability of albendazole, praziquantel and ivermectin combinations. *Transactions of the Royal Society of Tropical Medicine and Hygiene*, 2006, 100:335–345.

16. Ács N et al. Population-based case-control study of mebendazole in pregnant women for birth outcomes. *Congenital Anomalies*, 2005, 45:85–88.

17. de Silva NR et al. Effect of mebendazole therapy during pregnancy on birth outcome. *Lancet*, 1999, 353:1145–1149.

18. Diav-Citrin O et al. Pregnancy outcome after gestational exposure to mebendazole: a prospective controlled cohort study. *American Journal of Obstetrics and Gynecology*, 2003, 188:282–285.

19. Torlesse H, Hodges M. Anthelminthic treatment and haemoglobin concentrations during pregnancy. *Lancet*, 2000, 356:1083.

20. Torlesse H, Hodges M. Albendazole therapy and reduced decline in haemoglobin concentration during pregnancy (Sierra Leone). *Transactions of the Royal Society of Tropical Medicine and Hygiene*, 2001, 95:195–201.

21. Adam I, Elwasila ET, Homeida M. Is praziquantel therapy safe during pregnancy? *Transactions of the Royal Society of Tropical Medicine and Hygiene*, 2004, 98:540–543.

22. Pacque M et al. Pregnancy outcome after inadvertent ivermectin treatment during community-based distribution. *Lancet*, 1990, 336:1486–1489.

23. Chippaux JP et al. Absence of any adverse effect of inadvertent ivermectin treatment during pregnancy. *Transactions of the Royal Society of Tropical Medicine and Hygiene*, 1993, 87:318.

24. Gyapong JO et al. Treatment strategies underpinning the global programme to eliminate lymphatic filariasis. *Expert Opinion on Pharmacotherapeutics*, 2005, 6:179–200.

25. *Guidelines for drug donations*. Geneva, World Health Organization, 1999 (WHO/EDM/PAR/99.4).

26. *Guidelines for price discounts of single-source pharmaceuticals*. Geneva, World Health Organization, 2003 (WHO/EDM/PAR/2003.3).

27. Progress in measles control: Zambia, 1999–2004. *Weekly Epidemiological Record*, 2005, 80:213–217.

28. Centers for Disease Control and Prevention. Distribution of insecticide-treated bednets during an integrated nationwide immunization campaign – Togo, West Africa, December 2004. *Morbidity and Mortality Weekly Report*, 2004, 54:994–996.

29. Curtale F et al. Intestinal helminths and xerophthalmia in Nepal. A case-control study. *Journal of Tropical Pediatrics*, 1995, 41:334–337.

30. Mahalanabis D et al. Vitamin A absorption in ascariasis. *American Journal of Clinical Nutrition*, 1976, 29:1372–1375.

31. WHO/UNICEF. *How to add deworming to vitamin A distribution*. Geneva, World Health Organization, 2004 (WHO/CDS/CPE/PVC/2004.11).

32. *Community-directed treatment with ivermectin: report of a multi-country study*. Geneva, World Health Organization, 2006 (WHO/AFT/RP/96.1).

33. Montresor A et al. *Helminth control in school-age children. A guide for managers of control programmes*. Geneva, World Health Organization, 2002.

34. Ottesen EA. The Global Programme to Eliminate Lymphatic Filariasis. *Tropical Medicine and International Health*, 2000, 5:591–594.

35. Ottesen EA et al. Strategies and tools for the control/elimination of lymphatic filariasis. *Bulletin of the World Health Organization*, 1997, 75:491–503.

36. Ottesen EA, Ismail MM, Horton J. The role of albendazole in programmes to eliminate lymphatic filariasis. *Parasitology Today*, 1999, 15:382–386.

37. Sunish IP et al. Evidence for the use of albendazole for the elimination of lymphatic filariasis. *Lancet Infectious Diseases*, 2006, 6:125–126.

38. *Report of the First Meeting of the Technical Advisory Group on the Global Elimination of Lymphatic Filariasis.* Geneva, World Health Organization, 2000.

39. *Report of the Second Meeting of the Technical Advisory Group on the Global Elimination of Lymphatic Filariasis.* Geneva, World Health Organization, 2001.

40. *Report of the Fifth Meeting of the Technical Advisory Group on the Global Elimination of Lymphatic Filariasis.* Geneva, World Health Organization, 2004 (CDS/CPE/CEE/2004.42).

41. Remme J et al. Large scale ivermectin distribution and its epidemiological consequences. *Acta Leidensia*, 1990, 59:177–191.

42. Thylefors B, ed. Eliminating onchocerciasis as a public health problem. *Tropical Medicine and International Health*, 2004, 9(Suppl.):A1–A56.

43. Brieger WR et al. The effects of ivermectin on onchocercal skin disease and severe itching: results of a multicentre trial. *Tropical Medicine and International Health*, 1998, 3:951–961.

44. Burnham G. Ivermectin treatment of onchocercal skin lesions: observations from a placebo-controlled, double-blind trial in Malawi. *American Journal of Tropical Medicine and Hygiene*, 1995, 52:270–276.

45. Cousens SN et al. Impact of annual dosing with ivermectin on progression of onchocercal visual field loss. *Bulletin of the World Health Organization*, 1997, 75:229–236.

46. De Sole G et al. Adverse reactions after large-scale treatment of onchocerciasis with ivermectin: combined results from eight community trials. *Bulletin of the World Health Organization*, 1989, 67:707–719.

47. Boussinesq M, Prod'hon J, Chippaux JP. *Onchocerca volvulus*: striking decrease in transmission in the Vina valley (Cameroon) after eight annual large scale ivermectin treatments. *Transactions of the Royal Society of Tropical Medicine and Hygiene*, 1997, 91:82–86.

48. Cupp EW et al. The effects of repetitive community-wide ivermectin treatment on transmission of *Onchocerca volvulus* in Guatemala. *American Journal of Tropical Medicine and Hygiene*, 1992, 47:170–180.

49. Pacque M et al. Community-based treatment of onchocerciasis with ivermectin: safety, efficacy, and acceptability of yearly treatment. *Journal of Infectious Diseases*, 1991, 163:381–385.

50. *Strategies for ivermectin distribution through primary health care systems.* Geneva, World Health Organization, 1991 (WHO/PBL/91.24).

51. *Onchocerciasis and its control.* Report of a WHO Expert Committee on

Onchocerciasis Control. Geneva, World Health Organization, 1995 (WHO Technical Report Series, No. 852).

52. Crompton DWT et al., eds. Preparing to control schistosomiasis and soil-transmitted helminthiasis in the twenty-first century. *Acta Tropica*, 2003, 86:121–349.

53. *Prevention and control of schistosomiasis and soil-transmitted helminthiasis. Report of a WHO Expert Committee*. Geneva, World Health Organization, 2002 (WHO Technical Report Series, No. 912).

54. *Report of the WHO Informal Consultation on the use of praziquantel during pregnancy/lactation and albendazole/mebendazole in children under 24 months*. Geneva, World Health Organization, 2002 (WHO/CDS/CPE/PVC/2002.4).

55. Mehta DK, Ryan RSM, Hogerzeil HV, eds. *WHO Model Formulary 2004*. Geneva, World Health Organization, 2004.

56. Montresor A et al. Development and validation of a "tablet pole" for the administration of praziquantel in sub-Saharan Africa. *Transactions of the Royal Society of Tropical Medicine and Hygiene*, 2001, 95:542–544.

57. Montresor A et al. The WHO dose pole for the administration of praziquantel is also accurate in non-African populations. *Transactions of the Royal Society of Tropical Medicine and Hygiene*, 2005, 99:78–81.

58. Alexander ND et al. Ivermectin dose assessment without weighing scales. *Bulletin of the World Health Organization*, 1993, 71:361–366.

59. Pani SP, Das LK, Vanamail P. Tolerability and efficacy of a three-age class dosage schedule of diethylcarbamazine citrate (DEC) in the treatment of microfilaria carriers of *Wuchereria bancrofti* and its implications in mass drug administration (MDA) strategy for elimination of lymphatic filariasis (LF). *Journal of Communicable Diseases*, 2005, 37:12–17.

60. Savioli L, Crompton DWT, Neira M. Use of anthelminthic drugs during pregnancy. *American Journal of Obstetrics and Gynecology*, 2003, 188:5–6.

61. Christian P, Khatry SK, West KP Jr. Antenatal anthelminthic treatment, birthweight, and infant survival in rural Nepal. *Lancet*, 1994, 364:981–983.

62. Bradley M, Horton J. Assessing the risk of benzimidazole therapy during pregnancy. *Transactions of the Royal Society of Tropical Medicine and Hygiene*, 2001, 95:72–73.

63. *Report of the WHO Informal Consultation on hookworm infection and anaemia in girls and women*. Geneva, World Health Organization, 1996 (WHO/CTD/SIP/96.1).

64. Allen HE et al. New policies for using anthelminthics in high risk groups. *Trends in Parasitology*, 2002, 18:381–382.

65. Friedman JF, Kanzaria HK, McGarvey ST. Human schistosomiasis and anemia:

the relationship and potential mechanisms. *Trends in Parasitology*, 2005, 21:385–392.

66. Chippaux JP et al. Comparaison entre différentes méthodes de dépistage des grossesses au cours de traitements par ivermectine à large échelle au Cameroun [Comparison between various methods of pregnancy screening during a large-scale ivermectin treatment in Cameroon]. *Bulletin de la Société de Pathologie Exotique*, 1995, 88:129–133.

67. Gyapong JO, Chinbuah MA, Gyapong M. Inadvertent exposure of pregnant women to ivermectin and albendazole during mass drug administration for lymphatic filariasis. *Tropical Medicine and International Health*, 2003, 8:1093–1101.

68. Mectizan® Expert Committee/Technical Consultative Committee. *Recommendations for the treatment of onchocerciasis with Mectizan® in areas co-endemic for onchocerciasis and loiasis*, June 2004. Decatur, GA, Mectizan® Expert Committee/ Mectizan® Donation Program, 2004 (available at http://www.mectizan.org/library/EnglishMECTCCLoaRecs-June04.pdf; accessed 18 August 2006).

69. Mectizan® Expert Committee/Albendazole Coordination. *Report of 35th Meeting, London, United Kingdom, January 10–12, 2006*.

6. MEASURING AND MONITORING PREVENTIVE CHEMOTHERAPY

6.1 Coverage

Coverage is the minimum process indicator for assessing the performance of large-scale preventive chemotherapy interventions. In theory, coverage refers to the proportion of people in the target population or group who have actually swallowed the recommended drug or drug combinations. In practice, different approaches to determining and measuring coverage have been adopted in the field.

Before the start of a preventive chemotherapy intervention, the programme manager must define the target population (population eligible for treatment), calculate the number of doses required for each round of treatment, and develop a procedure for recording accurately the number of doses administered. A set of model forms for recording coverage rates is provided in Annex 5; these should be adapted by programme managers to suit the situations and environments in which they are working.

Every effort should be made to ensure direct observation of therapy (administration of the appropriate dose in the presence of the drug provider). If actual swallowing of tablets by targeted individuals cannot be observed directly, random cluster surveys – similar to those used to calculate the number of eligible children covered by the Expanded Programme on Immunization (EPI) – can be undertaken to estimate the actual coverage. If this approach is adopted, surveys for both preventive chemotherapy and EPI interventions could be conducted at the same time. Details of the methodology will be covered in a future manual on monitoring and evaluation of preventive chemotherapy interventions.

6.2 Evaluation of impact on morbidity and transmission

Target populations, health workers and community volunteers will lose interest in a preventive chemotherapy programme, especially in those communities where the infection reaches very low levels, unless regular information or bulletins are made available about the impact of the programme. Decision-makers may be more interested in the impact on morbidity (1). In programmes that target lymphatic filariasis and onchocerciasis, it is particularly important to also monitor impact on transmission of infection. Simple and measurable indicators applicable to each of the four helminthic diseases included in this manual are shown in Table 3. Detailed recommendations as to monitoring of impact will also be included in the separate manual on monitoring and evaluation of preventive chemotherapy interventions. Until this is available, preventive chemotherapy programmes should apply disease-

Table 3. Possible indicators for monitoring preventive chemotherapy interventions

Lymphatic filariasis	Onchocerciasis	Schistosomiasis	Soil-transmitted helminthiasis
Prevalence of microfilaraemia	Prevalence of onchocercal nodules	Prevalence of infection (by parasitological methods)	Prevalence of any infection (by parasitological methods)
Prevalence of antigenaemia	Prevalence of microfiladermia (skin snip test)	Intensity of infection (proportion of heavy-intensity infections)	Intensity of infection (proportion of heavy-intensity infections)
Prevalence of hydrocele		Prevalence of macrohaematuria	Prevalence of anaemia
Prevalence of lymphoedema		Prevalence of microhaematuria	
Incidence of acute attacks (adenolymphangitis)		Prevalence of anaemia	
Incidence of infection subsequent to MDA		Prevalence of ultrasound-detectable lesions (urinary tract and liver)	

specific procedures currently in use.

6.3 Threat of drug resistance and monitoring of drug efficacy

There is still little evidence of the emergence of drug resistance in human helminthiasis, but the problem is entrenched in helminths that infect livestock. Drug resistance should be suspected if high-coverage, high-frequency anthelminthic treatment is found to have less than the expected effect on the target helminths. Hookworms are known to be at higher risk than other helminths for developing drug resistance. Different resistance mechanisms and vector–host–parasite dynamics would play a role in the possible occurrence of reduced drug efficacy in lymphatic filariasis, onchocerciasis and schistosomiasis: the risk would be higher where the entire resident population was targeted, such as in interventions against lymphatic filariasis.

Long-term preventive chemotherapy must be accompanied by collection of baseline data on drug efficacy at the beginning of the intervention, followed by regular monitoring (*2, 3*). More detailed recommendations on how to monitor the threat of drug resistance will also be covered in the future manual on monitoring and evaluation of preventive chemotherapy interventions; until these become available, advice may be obtained from the World Health Organization (*4*).

References

1. *Report of the WHO Informal Consultation on the use of chemotherapy for the control of morbidity due to soil-transmitted nematodes in humans.* Geneva, World Health Organization, 1996 (WHO/CTD/SIP/96.2).

2. Geerts S, Gryseels B. Drug resistance in human helminths: current situation and lessons from livestock. *Clinical Microbiology Reviews*, 2000, 13:207–222.

3. Albonico M, Engels D, Savioli L. Monitoring drug efficacy and early detection of drug resistance in human soil-transmitted nematodes: a pressing public health agenda for helminth control. *International Journal of Parasitology*, 2004, 42:277–341.

4. *Report of the WHO Informal Consultation on monitoring of drug efficacy in the control of schistosomiasis and intestinal nematodes.* Geneva, World Health Organization, 1999 (WHO/CDS/CPC/SIP/99.1).

ANNEXES

Annex 1

Table 1. **Occurrence of lymphatic filariasis, onchocerciasis, schistosomiasis, soil-transmitted helminthiasis, and loiasis in countries and territories where preventive chemotherapy interventions may need to be implemented**

Country/territory	Lymphatic filariasis	Onchocerciasis	Schistosomiasis	Soil-transmitted helminthiasis	Loa-loa[a]
WHO African Region					
Algeria				✓	
Angola	✓	✓	✓	✓	✓
Benin	✓	✓	✓	✓	
Botswana	✓		✓	✓	
Burkina Faso	✓	✓	✓	✓	
Burundi	✓	✓	✓	✓	✓
Cameroon	✓	✓	✓	✓	✓
Cape Verde	✓			✓	
Central African Republic	✓	✓	✓	✓	✓
Chad	✓	✓	✓	✓	✓
Comoros	✓			✓	
Congo	✓	✓	✓	✓	✓
Côte d'Ivoire	✓	✓	✓	✓	
Democratic Republic of the Congo	✓	✓	✓	✓	✓
Equatorial Guinea	✓	✓	✓	✓	✓
Eritrea			✓	✓	✓
Ethiopia	✓	✓	✓	✓	✓
Gabon	✓	✓	✓	✓	✓
Gambia	✓		✓	✓	
Ghana	✓	✓	✓	✓	✓
Guinea	✓	✓	✓	✓	
Guinea-Bissau	✓	✓	✓	✓	✓
Kenya	✓	✓	✓	✓	
Lesotho				✓	
Liberia	✓	✓	✓	✓	
Madagascar	✓		✓	✓	
Malawi	✓	✓	✓	✓	
Mali	✓	✓	✓	✓	
Mauritania			✓	✓	
Mauritius	✓			✓	
Mozambique	✓	✓	✓	✓	
Namibia	✓		✓	✓	
Niger	✓	✓	✓	✓	✓
Nigeria	✓	✓	✓	✓	✓
Rwanda	✓	✓	✓	✓	
SaoTome and Principe	✓		✓	✓	
Senegal	✓	✓	✓	✓	
Seychelles	✓			✓	

Country/territory	Lymphatic filariasis	Onchocerciasis	Schistosomiasis	Soil-transmitted helminthisasis	Loa-loa[a]
Sierra Leone	✓	✓	✓	✓	✔
South Africa			✓	✓	
Swaziland			✓	✓	
Togo	✓	✓	✓	✓	
Uganda	✓	✓	✓	✓	✔
United Republic of Tanzania	✓	✓	✓	✓	
Zambia	✓		✓	✓	
Zimbabwe	✓		✓	✓	

WHO Region of the Americas

Country/territory	Lymphatic filariasis	Onchocerciasis	Schistosomiasis	Soil-transmitted helminthisasis	Loa-loa[a]
Antigua and Barbuda				✓	
Bahamas				✓	
Barbados				✓	
Belize				✓	
Bolivia				✓	
Brazil	✓	✓	✓	✓	
Colombia		✓		✓	
Costa Rica	✓[b]			✓	
Cuba				✓	
Dominica				✓	
Dominican Republic	✓		✓	✓	
Ecuador		✓		✓	
El Salvador				✓	
Grenada				✓	
Guatemala		✓		✓	
Guyana	✓			✓	
Haiti	✓			✓	
Honduras				✓	
Jamaica				✓	
Mexico		✓		✓	
Nicaragua				✓	
Panama				✓	
Paraguay				✓	
Peru				✓	
Puerto Rico				✓	
Saint Kitts and Nevis				✓	
Saint Lucia				✓	
Saint Vincent and the Grenadines				✓	
Suriname			✓	✓	
Trinidad and Tobago				✓	
Venezuela		✓	✓	✓	

Country/territory	Lymphatic filariasis	Onchocerciasis	Schistosomiasis	Soil-transmitted helminthisasis	Loa-loa[a]
WHO Eastern Mediterranean Region					
Afghanistan				✓	
Bahrain					
Djibouti				✓	
Egypt	✓		✓	✓	
Iran (Islamic Republic of)				✓	
Iraq			✓	✓	
Jordan					
Libyan Arab Jamahiriya					
Morocco					
Oman					
Pakistan				✓	
Palestine				✓	
Qatar					
Saudi Arabia					
Somalia			✓	✓	
Sudan	✓	✓	✓	✓	✓
Syrian Arab Republic					
Tunisia					
Yemen	✓	✓	✓	✓	
WHO South-East Asia Region					
Bangladesh	✓			✓	
Bhutan				✓	
Dem. People's Republic of Korea				✓	
India	✓			✓	
Indonesia	✓			✓	
Maldives	✓			✓	
Myanmar	✓			✓	
Nepal	✓			✓	
Sri Lanka	✓			✓	
Thailand	✓			✓	
Timor-Leste	✓			✓	

Country/territory	Lymphatic filariasis	Onchocerciasis	Schistosomiasis	Soil-transmitted helminthisasis	Loa-loa[a]
WHO Western Pacific Region					
Brunei Darussalam	✓				
Cambodia	✓		✓	✓	
China	✓[b]		✓	✓	
Cook Islands	✓			✓	
Fiji	✓			✓	
Kiribati	✓			✓	
Lao PDR	✓[b]		✓	✓	
Malaysia	✓			✓	
Marshall Islands	✓			✓	
Micronesia (Federated States of)	✓			✓	
Nauru				✓	
Niue	✓			✓	
Palau				✓	
Papua New Guinea	✓			✓	
Philippines	✓		✓	✓	
Republic of Korea	✓[b]				
Samoa	✓			✓	
Singapore					
Solomon Islands	✓[b]			✓	
Tokelau				✓	
Tonga	✓			✓	
Tuvalu	✓			✓	
Vanuatu	✓			✓	
Viet Nam	✓			✓	
American Samoa[c]	✓			✓	
French Polynesia[c]	✓			✓	
New Caledonia[c]	✓			✓	
Wallis and Futuna[c]	✓			✓	

[a] This is a provisional list. Mapping activities for *Loa loa* are still in progress and other countries may prove to be endemic.
[b] Recent mapping surveys have indicated the possibility of there being no active transmission of lymphatic filariasis in these countries.
[c] Territories.

Rapid assessment and decision charts for schistosomiasis and soil-transmitted helminthiasis

Step 1: Epidemiological survey

Sampling for soil-transmitted helminthiasis

Divide the country or district in ecologicaly homogeneous areas and consider for rapid assessment those where STH transmission is suspected. Choose 5–10 schools in each area. In each school, select 50 children from any of the three upper classes (where the infection rates will be the highest). Take a stool sample from each child and examine it for presence and number of soil-transmitted helminth eggs using the Kato–Katz method. In the same sample you will also see the eggs of intestinal schistosomes if they are present.

Sampling for schistosomiasis

The schools you choose for soil-transmitted helminthiasis may be in areas that are free of schistosomiasis (which is found only around water). To survey for schistosomiasis, you need to survey specifically some areas that are near lakes, ponds, streams or irrigated areas. First, try to find any old surveys, which will give you an idea of whether schistosomiasis has been identified in a particular locality or area in the past. Then consult health services data which are often the best source of information. If schistosomiasis is suspected, select a few schools close to the water and some a little further away and investigate as follows:

For intestinal schistosomiasis.

From each school you have chosen, select 50 children from the upper classes and ask each of them to provide a stool sample. Using the Kato–Katz method, examine the samples for presence and number of intestinal schistosome eggs.

For urinary schistosomiasis.

Select the schools in the same way. You then have the choice of two methods to assess the magnitude of the problem. The simplest approach is to use the standard questionnaire for visible haematuria: send 50 questionnaires to each school (one per child in the upper classes). Questionnaires can also be used to assess population outside schools. Alternative methods are: assessment of visible and macrohaematuria and/or the use of a urine filtration kit to examine a urine sample for presence and number of schistosome eggs from each of the 50 children selected from the upper classes of each school.

Step 2: Making a plan

Since the stool and urine samples are analysed on the day of the survey, it should not take long to collate the results and produce a short report that describes the prevalence and intensity of infection in each school and each area. A software for the input of each child's age, parasitological data, height, weight and haemoglobin, during a survey is available at: http://www.who.int/wormcontrol/documents/software/en/. The following tables should then be used to determine the appropriate action.

Table A2.1 **Recommended treatment strategy for STH in preventive chemotherapy[a]**

Category	Prevalence of any STH infection among school-aged children	Action to be taken	
High-risk community	≥50%	Treat all school-age children (enrolled and not enrolled) twice each year[b]	Also treat: <ul><li>preschool children;</li><li>women of childbearing age, including pregnant women in the 2nd and 3rd trimesters and lactating women;</li><li>adults at high risk in certain occupations (e.g. tea-pickers and miners)</li></ul>
Low-risk community	≥20% and <50%	Treat all school-age children (enrolled and not enrolled) once each year	Also treat: <ul><li>preschool children;</li><li>women of childbearing age, including pregnant women in the 2nd and 3rd trimesters and lactating women;</li><li>adults at high risk in certain occupations (e.g. tea-pickers and miners)</li></ul>

[a] When prevalence of any STH infection is less than 20%, large-scale preventive chemotherapy interventions are not recommended. Affected individuals should be dealt with on a case-by-case basis.
[b] If resources are available, a third drug distribution intervention might be added. In this case the appropriate frequency of treatment would be every 4 months.

Table A2.2 **Recommended treatment strategy for schistosomiasis in preventive chemotherapy**

Category	Prevalence among school-aged children	Action to be taken	
High-risk community	≥50% by parasitological methods (intestinal and urinary schistosomiasis) or ≥30% by questionnaire for visible haematuria (urinary schistosomiasis)	Treat all school-age children (enrolled and not enrolled) once a year	Also treat adults considered to be at risk (from special groups to entire communities living in endemic areas; see Annex 6 for details on special groups)
Moderate-risk community	≥10% but <50% by parasitological methods (intestinal and urinary schistosomiasis) or <30% by questionnaire for visible haematuria (urinary schistosomiasis)	Treat all school-age children (enrolled and not enrolled) once every 2 years	Also treat adults considered to be at risk (special risk groups only; see Annex 6 for details on special groups)
Low-risk community	<10% by parasitological methods (intestinal and urinary schistosomiasis)	Treat all school-age children (enrolled and not enrolled) twice during their primary schooling age (e.g. once on entry and once on exit)	Praziquantel should be available in dispensaries and clinics for treatment of suspected cases

Standardized form for recording serious adverse experiences

SERIOUS ADVERSE EXPERIENCE REPORTING FORM

For programmes in which one or more anthelminthic drugs (including albendazole, DEC, ivermectin, mebendazole, and praziquantel) are used in large-scale interventions against intestinal helminthiasis, lymphatic filariasis, onchocerciasis, and/or schistosomiasis, the following form should be used.

A **serious adverse experience (SAE)** is defined as an adverse experience following treatment with a drug that results in any of the following:

- death
- life-threatening condition
- in-patient hospitalization or prolongation of an existing hospitalization
- persistent or significant disability/incapacity
- congenital anomaly or birth defect
- cancer
- overdose (accidental or intentional).

Important medical events that may not result in death, be life-threatening, or require hospitalization may be considered as SAEs when, based upon appropriate medical judgement, they may jeopardize the patient or subject, and may require medical or surgical intervention to prevent one of the outcomes listed in the definition above: such events should also be reported.

Complete this form only if the adverse experience meets the above criteria and send it promptly to:

Drugs	Contacts	
All drugs used in all interventions	Responsible Officer for Pharmacovigilance Quality Assurance and Safety of Medicines (QSM) Department of Medicines Policy and Standards (PSM) World Health Organization Avenue Appia 20 1211 Geneva 27, Switzerland	Telephone: + 41 22 791 3643/12337 Fax: + 41 22 791 4761 E-mail: couperm@who.int orscudamorec@who.int
Mectizan® (ivermectin) is donated by Merck & Co., Inc for lymphatic filariasis elimination and onchocerciasis control programmes	Mectizan® Donation Program* 750 Commerce Drive, Ste. 400 Decatur, GA 30030 USA * Receives SAEs on behalf of Merck & Co., Inc.	Telephone: +1 404 371 1460 Fax: +1 404 371 1138 E-mail: mectizan@taskforce.org
Albendazole donated by GlaxoSmithKline for lymphatic filariasis elimination programmes	Global Clinical Safety & Pharmacovigilance GlaxoSmithKline Essex England	Telephone: +44 1279 644174 Fax: +44 20 8966 2338 E-mail: OAX37649@gsk.com
Mebendazole donated by Johnson and Johnson Pharmaceutical for soil-transmitted helminths control programmes	BRM Case Management Centre Johnson & Johnson Pharmaceuticals 50-100 Holmers Farm Way High Wycombe Bucks. HP12 4DP United Kingdom	Telephone: +44 1494 658952 Fax: +44 1494 658273

Country:	Date of report: / / (day/month/year)

1. Patient information

Name (first/middle/last)		**Age** (years)	**Sex** (M/F)
Location	District	Province/State	

2. Pre-existing conditions

Health status before treatment with the drugs:

☐ Good ☐ Poor ☐ Unknown   If "Poor", give details:

Parasitic infections	Confirmed	Suspected	Negative	Unknown	Details
1. STH ⇒	☐	☐	☐	☐	
2. Lymphatic filariasis ⇒	☐	☐	☐	☐	
3. Onchocerciasis ⇒	☐	☐	☐	☐	
4. Schistosomiasis ⇒	☐	☐	☐	☐	

Other parasitic infections, known or suspected:

Malaria   ☐ Yes   ☐ No

Loiasis   ☐ Yes   ☐ No   ⇒   If "Yes", mf/ml (blood):   mf/ml (CSF):

Other medications being taken (currently or recently):

Is patient pregnant? ☐ Yes   ☐ No   ☐ Unknown

3. Drugs administered

Which of the following drugs were administered to the patient? (check all that apply) | Date of treatment: (day/month/year)

☐ albendazole   ⇒   /   /

☐ diethylcarbamazine (DEC)   ⇒   /   /

☐ ivermectin   ⇒   /   /

☐ mebendazole   ⇒   /   /

☐ praziquantel   ⇒   /   /

Source of treatment: ☐ Mass treatment programme ☐ Clinic or physician treatment ☐ Other method	*Patient's height* (cm) ⇓	*Patient's weight* (kg) ⇓

Dose of albendazole no. and strength of tablets	Dose of DEC no. and strength of tablets	Dose of ivermectin no. and strength of tablets	Dose of mebendazole no. and strength of tablets	Dose of praziquantel no. and strength of tablets
Manufacturer name if available	Manufacturer name if available	Manufacturer name if available	Manufacturer name if available	Manufacturer name if available
Batch number if available	Batch number if available	Batch number if available	Batch number if available	Batch number if available

Was this a first treatment with any of the drugs selected above?

☐ Yes   ☐ No   ☐ Unknown

If "Yes", which of the following drugs were first treatments?

☐ albendazole   ☐ diethylcarbamazine (DEC)   ☐ ivermectin   ☐ mebendazole   ☐ praziquantel

If "No", explain when, and circumstances of past treatment(s) of each drug:

4. Description of the serious adverse experience (SAE)

Date of onset (day/month/year) / /	How long after drugs were taken? hours OR days

Clinical signs and symptoms (please describe)

Do you think this adverse experience is/was life-threatening?   ☐ Yes ☐ No

Laboratory results (please provide name of test)   Dates of tests (day/month/year)

⇒   /   /

⇒   /   /

⇒   /   /

a*) Hospitalization*   ☐ Yes   ☐ No

    If "Yes", indicate: 1. Date of admission (day/month/year) ⇒   /   /

                     2. Reason for admission:

                     3. Date of discharge (day/month/year) ⇒   /   /

b) *Drug treatments administered:*

c) *Clinical course:*

(Attach any relevant reports)

5. Condition/outcome at time of last observation

Full recovery: ☐ Yes   ☐ No   ☐ Unknown

Ongoing illness: ☐ Yes   ☐ No   ☐ Unknown

    If "Yes", describe current condition:

Persistent/significant disability/incapacity: ☐ Yes   ☐ No   ☐ Unknown

    If "Yes", describe:

Death: ☐ Yes   ☐ No

      If "Yes", indicate: 1.   Date of death (day/month/year):   /   /

                      2.   Cause of death:

                      3.   Circumstances at the time of death, in detail:

      Report any autopsy findings, including tissues taken for histopathology and any additional studies done or requested (use additional pages if necessary to complete your answers):

---

6. Conclusions (to be completed by the health-care provider)

Presumptive diagnosis:

Do you think the combined treatment with the drugs selected in Box 3 was a possible causative factor in this serious adverse experience?

     ☐ Yes   ☐ No   ☐ Not sure

     If "Yes", explain:

     If "No" or "Not sure", what do you believe was the cause of the experience?

7. Source (reporter(s) of the data in this form)	
Name of person making the report $\Rightarrow$	
Title $\Rightarrow$	
Organization $\Rightarrow$	
Address $\Rightarrow$	
Telephone number $\Rightarrow$	
Fax number $\Rightarrow$	

Annex 4

Drug supply, recommended dosages and dose poles

Albendazole is donated by GlaxoSmithKline for as long as necessary to achieve elimination of lymphatic filariasis as a public health problem, and ivermectin (Mectizan®) by Merck and Co., Inc., for elimination of lymphatic filariasis and control of onchocerciasis.

Generic albendazole or mebendazole need to be procured where:
- LF is not endemic and STH are endemic;
- LF and STH are both endemic, but a single annual drug distribution with albendazole for LF is not sufficient for the control of STH.

The average market price of a single tablet of generic albendazole (400mg) or mebendazole (500mg) is around US$ 0.02–0.03.

Where lymphatic filariasis is not endemic, albendazole is not donated and therefore needs to be procured: the current lowest price of a generic 400-mg tablet is US$ 0.02.

Although DEC is not donated, it is available from several manufacturers at low cost (around US$ 4.00 for a box of 1000 tablets).

Praziquantel is not donated and the current lowest price of a generic 600-mg tablet is approximately US$ 0.08.

Drugs that are not donated can be procured as generics by national or international producers through the national procurement service. WHO can also provide help and guidance. To obtain assistance with procurement of drugs and other material, please contact the Office of the WHO Representative in your country through your Ministry of Health.

Recommended doses of the various drugs are given in Table A4.1; the dose poles for use in large-scale administration of praziquantel and ivermectin are illustrated in Figure A4.1.

Table A4.1 Recommended drugs and dosages in preventive chemotherapy interventions

	Age/height	ALB	MBD	LEV	PYR	DEC[a]	IVM[b]	PZQ[c]
By age group	12–23 months	200 mg	500 mg	2.5 mg/kg	10 mg/kg	–		
	2–5 years	400 mg	500 mg	2.5 mg/kg	10 mg/kg	1 tablet (100 mg)		
	6–15 years	400 mg	500 mg	2 tablets[d] (80 mg)	10 mg/kg	2 tablets (200 mg)		
	>15 years	400 mg	500 mg	2.5 mg/kg	10 mg/kg	3 tablets (300 mg)		
By height	90–119 cm						1 tablet (3 mg)	
	120–139 cm						2 tablets (6 mg)	
	141–159 cm						3 tablets (9 mg)	
	>159 cm						4 tablets (12 mg)	
	94–109 cm							1 tablet (600 mg)
	110–124 cm							1½ tablets (900 mg)
	125–137 cm							2 tablets (1200 mg)
	138–149 cm							2 ½ tablets (1500 mg)
	150–159 cm							3 tablets (1800 mg)
	160–177 cm							4 tablets (2400 mg)
	≥178 cm							5 tablets (3000 mg)

[a] Using 100-mg DEC tablets.
[b] Using 3-mg IVM tablets.
[c] Using 600-mg PZQ tablets.
[d] Using 40-mg LEV tablets.

Figure A4.1 Recommended dose-poles for large-scale administration of PZQ (600 mg tablet) and IVM (3 mg tablet)

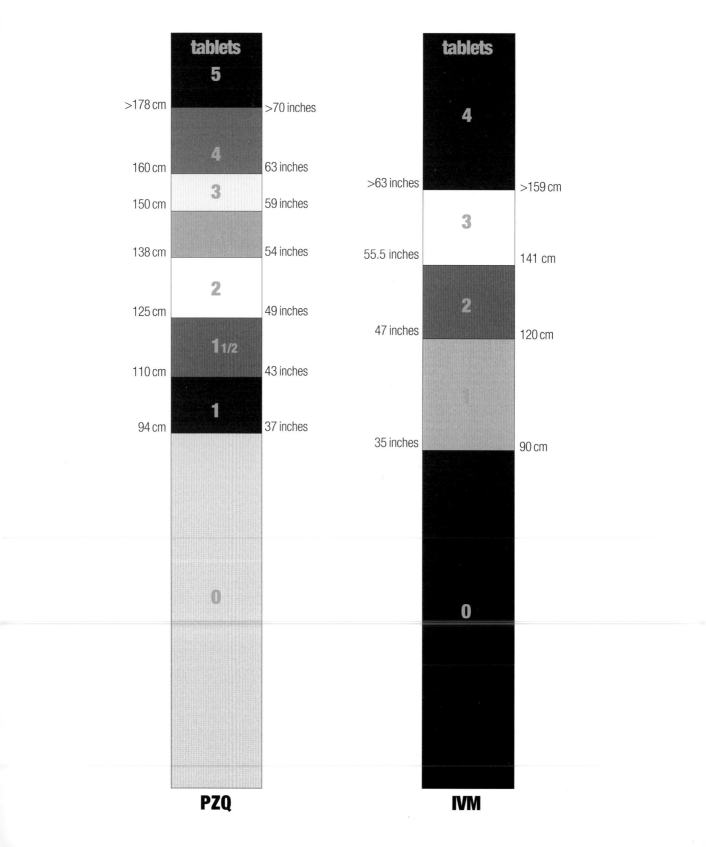

Coverage forms

The following forms are proposed for recording the coverage achieved during preventive chemotherapy interventions. Programme managers should adapt them as necessary in the context of their working environment. Two sets of forms are available according to the selected interventions: the first set is designed for use in mass drug administration interventions (MDA1, MDA2, MDA3), the second set for targeted treatment interventions (T1, T2, T3). Each set has two forms – one for the sub-district level and one for district-level compilation.

First set – to be used in MDA1, MDA2, MD3 interventions.
    Drugs used: IVM+ALB or DEC+ALB or IVM only
    Form 1: sub-district level compilation
    Form 2: district-level compilation

Note: For appropriate calculation of coverage, cross out the ALB column on Forms 1 and 2 if ALB is not distributed (i.e. in MDA3 interventions).

Second set – to be used in T1, T2, T3 interventions
    Drugs used: PZQ and/or ALB/MBD
    Form 3: sub-district level compilation
    Form 4: district-level compilation

Note: For appropriate calculation of coverage, cross out the ALB/MBD column on Forms 3 and 4 if there is no distribution of ALB or MBD (i.e. in T2 interventions); similarly, cross out the PZQ column if PZQ is not distributed (i.e. in T3 interventions).

Form 1: for village/urban area/school/health post recording of drug coverage (MDA1, MDA2, MDA3)

Region:		Village/urban area/school/health post:	
District:		Campaign/round of treatment:	
Date:		Drugs distributed:	

Class/household/ treatment point	Total population	Eligible population	Number of individuals ingesting an appropriate dose of treatment [cross out the ALB column in MDA3 interventions]	
			ALB	IVM/DEC
1				
2				
3				
4				
5				
6				
7				
8				
9				
10				
11				
12				
13				
14				
15				
16				
17				
18				
19				
20				
21				
22				
23				
24				
25				
26				
27				
28				
29				
30				

Total by village/urban area/school/health post:

Village/ urban area/ school/ health post	(A) Total population	(B) Eligible population	No. of individuals ingesting an appropriate dose of treatment:		Reported coverage	
			(C) ALB	(D) IVM/DEC	% of total population (D/A) x 100	% of eligible population (D/B) x 100

Form 2: for district reporting of drug coverage (MDA1, MDA2, MDA3)							
Region:		Campaign/round of treatment:					
District:							
Date:		Drugs distributed:					
Total number of urban areas in district:		Total number of villages in district:					
Number of urban areas covered:		Number of villages covered:					

Village/ urban area/ school/ health post	Targeted for ONCHO (Y/N)	Total population	Eligible population	Number of individuals ingesting an appropriate dose of treatment [cross out the ALB column in MDA3 interventions]		Reported drug coverage	
				ALB	IVM/DEC	% of total population	% of eligible population
1							
2							
3							
4							
5							
6							
7							
8							
9							
10							
11							
12							
13							
14							
15							
16							
17							
18							
19							
20							
21							
22							
23							
24							
25							
26							
27							
28							
29							
30							

Total by district:

District	(A) Total population	(B) Eligible population	Number of individuals ingesting an appropriate dose of treatment		Reported coverage	
			(C) ALB	(D) IVM/DEC	% of total population (D/A) x 100	% of eligible population (D/B) x 100

Form 3: for village/urban area/school/health post recording of drug coverage (T1, T2, T3)					
Region:			Village/urban area/school/health post:		
District:			Campaign/round of treatment:		
Date:			Drugs distributed:		
Class/ household/ treatment point	Number of eligible individuals	Number of targeted individuals	Number of targeted individuals ingesting an appropriate dose of treatment: [cross out the ALB/MBD column in T2 interventions; cross out the PZQ column in T3 interventions]		
			ALB/MBD	PZQ	
1					
2					
3					
4					
5					
6					
7					
8					
9					
10					
11					
12					
13					
14					
15					
16					
17					
18					
19					
20					
21					
22					
23					
24					
25					
26					
27					
28					
29					
30					
Total by village/urban area/school/health post:					
Village/urban area/school/ health post	Number of eligible individuals	Number of targeted individuals	Number of targeted individuals ingesting an appropriate dose of treatment		Coverage (%)
			ALB/MBD	PZQ	

Form 4: for district recording of drug coverage (T1, T2, T3)				
Region:				
District:		Campaign/round of treatment:		
Date:		Drugs distributed:		
Village/ urban area/ school/ health post	Number of targeted individuals	Number of targeted individuals ingesting an appropriate dose of treatment: [cross out the ALB/MBD column in T2 interventions; cross out the PZQ column in T3 interventions		Coverage (%)
		ALB/MBD	PZQ	
1				
2				
3				
4				
5				
6				
7				
8				
9				
10				
11				
12				
13				
14				
15				
16				
17				
18				
19				
20				
21				
22				
23				
24				
25				
26				
27				
28				
29				
30				
Total by district:				
District	Number of targeted individuals	Number of targeted individuals receiving an appropriate dose of treatment		Coverage %
		ALB/MBD	PZQ	

Annex 6

Disease-specific information

A6.1 Lymphatic filariasis

The disease
It is estimated that 1.2 billion people in 83 countries live in areas endemic for lymphatic filariasis and about 120 million people are affected by the disease.

The causal agents of lymphatic filariasis are the filariae *Wuchereria bancrofti, Brugia malayi* and *Brugia timori*. The adult worms live in the lymphatic system of humans. After mating, each female worm produces several thousand larvae (microfilariae), which appear in the peripheral blood at times that coincide with the biting activity of mosquito vectors. The microfilariae are ingested along with the blood meal by the mosquitoes, develop inside the insects and are transmitted to another human host through mosquito bites.

Filarial infection may be clinically asymptomatic; the disease may also present as one or more acute manifestations (fever, local swelling, tropical pulmonary eosinophilia syndrome, lymphangitis). Chronic complications include lymphoedema or elephantiasis of the limbs, damage to the genital organs (including hydrocele in men), and damage to the kidney (including chyluria) and lymphatic system.

Recommended intervention strategy and aim
The strategy of the Global Programme to Eliminate Lymphatic Filariasis has two components:

- Mass drug administration of two drugs (DEC + albendazole or ivermectin + albendazole), given together to the entire eligible population once a year until transmission is reduced and ultimately interrupted, or regular intake of DEC-fortified salt.
- Home-based care to prevent and alleviate the suffering of affected individuals and community education programmes to promote the benefits of intensive local hygiene and self-management of affected organs and limbs.

Eligible population
The entire population at risk of lymphatic filariasis transmission, i.e. the entire population in an area where transmission occurs (implementation unit), except those excluded (see ineligible population).

Ineligible population
In areas where ivermectin and albendazole are used: pregnant women, lactating women in the first week after birth, children under 90 cm in height (approximately equivalent to a weight of 15 kg), and the severely ill.

In areas where DEC and albendazole are used: pregnant women, children under 2 years of age, and the severely ill.

Access to drugs

Albendazole is donated by GlaxoSmithKline and ivermectin (Mectizan®) by Merck and Co., Inc., for as long as necessary to ensure success of the elimination programme. Although DEC is not donated, it is available at low cost from several manufacturers.

World Health Assembly targets and deadlines

Resolution WHA50.29 (1997) urged Member States "…to take advantage of recent advances in the understanding of lymphatic filariasis and the new opportunities for its elimination by developing national plans…" and "…to improve clinical, epidemiological and operational activities directed towards eliminating lymphatic filariasis as a public health problem".

Web site

http://www.who.int/neglected_diseases/diseases/en/
or
http://www.who.int/lymphatic_filariasis/en/

A6.2 Onchocerciasis (river blindness)

The disease

Onchocerciasis is endemic in 30 countries in Africa, 6 countries in the Americas, and in Yemen in the Arabian peninsula. In 1995 it was estimated that 17.7 million people were infected, of whom 268 000 were considered to be blind as a result of the disease; more recent data, however, indicate that these figures were largely underestimated. There has been a significant reduction in the extent and public health significance of onchocerciasis in the countries included in the Onchocerciasis Control Programme (see below): most of the problem now is to be found in the African countries that were not included in the Programme. Today, more than 99% of those infected live in Africa.

The causal agent of onchocerciasis is *Onchocerca volvulus*, a nematode filaria. The adult worm lives in the human body in fibrous, subcutaneous nodules. Each adult female produces millions of microfilariae that migrate under the skin and through the eyes, giving rise to a variety of dermal and ocular symptoms. The vector for onchocerciasis is the blackfly (genus *Simulium*), whose larvae live in fast-running waters – this has led to the name "river blindness". The female blackfly may ingest microfilariae by taking a blood meal from an infected person. Microfilariae transform into infective larvae within the blackfly after several days; they are then injected into the person from whom the next blood meal is taken and subsequently develop into adult parasites.

Symptoms begin 1–3 years after infection, usually at the time when adult females begin to produce microfilariae. These include: rashes, papular skin lesions, subcutaneous nodules, intense itching and depigmentation of the skin, lymphadenitis, which results in "hanging groin" and elephantiasis of the genitalia, and general debilitation. Eye lesions lead to serious visual impairment including blindness.

Recommended intervention strategy and aim

Yearly distribution of ivermectin to meso- and hyperendemic communities is the standard option. However, drug distribution may take place more frequently: in some countries, the national plans recommend treatment every 6 months (aiming at controlling morbidity and eventually interrupting transmission).

Control activities are organized on a regional basis as outlined in the following paragraphs:

Onchocerciasis Control Programme (OCP). OCP was launched in 1974 and officially closed in 2002. Its goal was to eliminate onchocerciasis as a public health problem and an obstacle to socioeconomic development from 11 west African countries. Vector control was the main strategy – and the only strategy from 1974 to 1988. From 1988 (when the Mectizan® Donation Program was established) until 2002, vector control was coupled with mass distribution of ivermectin. Vector control is continuing in five countries (Benin, Ghana, Guinea, Sierra Leone and Togo) of the former OCP, known as Special Intervention Zones. In all the 11 countries, detection of transmission recrudescence and disease control through IVM distribution are now routine functions of national disease surveillance and control services.

African Programme for Onchocerciasis Control (APOC). APOC's goal is to eliminate onchocerciasis as a disease of public health importance and an important constraint on socioeconomic development in 19 African countries. Community-directed treatment with ivermectin (CDTI) is the main strategy of APOC, coupled with vector control in four selected foci in Equatorial Guinea (1 focus), United Republic of Tanzania (1 focus) and Uganda (2 foci).

Onchocerciasis Elimination Program for the Americas (OEPA). The goal of OEPA is elimination of onchocerciasis as a public health problem, defined as elimination of morbidity – and interruption of transmission where feasible – in six endemic countries in the Americas (Brazil, Colombia, Ecuador, Guatemala, Mexico and Venezuela) through mass treatment with ivermectin.

Eligible population

The entire population in meso- and hyperendemic communities (where prevalence of infection – i.e. prevalence of positive skin snips – is ≥40% or prevalence of palpable nodules is ≥20%), except those excluded (see ineligible population).

Ineligible population

Pregnant women, lactating women in the first week after birth, children under 90 cm in height (approximately equivalent to a weight of 15 kg), and the severely ill.

Access to drugs

Ivermectin (Mectizan®) is donated by Merck and Co., Inc., to endemic countries through the Mectizan Donation Program for the treatment of onchocerciasis, to all who need it for as long as needed.

World Health Assembly targets and deadlines

Resolution WHA47.32 (1994) requested Member States "…to prepare national plans…for the control of onchocerciasis through vector control, where applicable, and the regular distribution of ivermectin to populations in need…". Target dates for OEPA (elimination) and APOC (elimination as a public health problem) are currently 2007 and 2010, respectively.

Partnerships

Vision 2020: The Right to Sight is a global initiative of the International Agency for the Prevention of Blindness and WHO, with a coalition of international nongovernmental organizations. It aims to eliminate unnecessary blindness in order to give all people in the world, particularly the millions of needlessly blind, the right to sight; onchocerciasis is one of the diseases it is concerned with.

More specifically on onchocerciasis, the NGDO Group for Onchocerciasis Control groups together WHO, APOC, OEPA, the ministries of health of endemic countries, and several nongovernmental development organizations (NGDOs). Regular meetings are held.

Web site

http://www.who.int/neglected_diseases/diseases/en/
or
http://www.who.int/topics/onchocerciasis/en/

A6.3 Schistosomiasis

The disease

Schistosomiasis affects about 200 million people worldwide, and more than 650 million people live in endemic areas. Urinary schistosomiasis is caused by *Schistosoma haematobium* and intestinal schistosomiasis by any of the organisms *S. intercalatum*, *S. mansoni*, *S. japonicum*, and *S. mekongi*. Several million people all over the world suffer from severe morbidity as a consequence of schistosomiasis.

Causal agents of the disease are fluke worms (schistosomes). Their eggs leave the human body in urine (in urinary schistosomiasis) or faeces (in intestinal schistosomiasis), hatch in water and liberate larvae (miracidia) that penetrate into freshwater snail hosts. After several weeks, cercariae emerge from the snails and penetrate the human skin (during wading, swimming, washing). Cercariae develop to maturity within the body and subsequently migrate to the lungs, the liver, and the veins of the abdominal cavity or the bladder plexus. Eggs escape through the bowel or urinary bladder.

Disease is caused primarily by schistosome eggs, which are deposited by adult worms in the blood vessels surrounding the bladder or intestines. The classical sign of *urinary schistosomiasis* is haematuria (blood in urine). Bladder and ureteral fibrosis and hydronephrosis are common findings in advanced cases, and bladder cancer is also a possible late-stage complications. *Intestinal schistosomiasis* has a nonspecific clinical picture of abdominal pain, diarrhoea, and blood in the stool. Liver enlargement is common in advanced cases and frequently associated with ascites and other signs of increased portal pressure. In such cases there may also be splenomegaly.

Recommended intervention strategy and aim

Targeted distribution of praziquantel is the norm. Intervention frequency is determined by the prevalence of infection or of visible haematuria (for *S. haematobium* only) among school-age children (see Annex 2). The aim is morbidity control: periodic treatment of at-risk populations will cure subtle morbidity and prevent infected individuals from developing severe, late-stage morbidity due to schistosomiasis.

Eligible population

- School-age children.
- Adults considered to be at risk, from special groups (pregnant and lactating women; groups with occupations involving contact with infested water, such as fishermen, farmers, irrigation workers, or women in their domestic tasks), to entire communities living in endemic areas.

Ineligible population

There is no documented information on the safety of praziquantel for children under 4 years of age (or under 94 cm in height). These children should therefore be excluded from large-scale preventive chemotherapy interventions but can be treated on an individual basis by medical personnel.

Access to drugs

Praziquantel is not donated. The cost of a single 600-mg tablets is about US$ 0.08 and of an average treatment is about US$ 0.20–0.30.

World Health Assembly targets and deadlines

Resolution WHA54.19 (2001) urged Member States "…to ensure access to essential drugs against schistosomiasis…in all health services in endemic areas for the treatment of clinical cases and groups at high risk of morbidity such as women and children, with the goal of attaining a minimum target of regular administration of chemotherapy to at least 75% and up to 100% of all school-age children at risk of morbidity by 2010".

Web site

http://www.who.int/neglected_diseases/diseases/en/

The disease

Soil-transmitted helminthiasis affects more than 2000 million people worldwide. The causal agent of soil-transmitted helminthiasis is any of the following worms: *Ascaris lumbricoides*, *Trichuris trichiura* and the hookworms. Recent estimates[1] suggest that *Ascaris lumbricoides* infects 1.221 billion people, *Trichuris trichiura* 795 million, and hookworms (*Ancylostoma duodenale* and *Necator americanus*) 740 million. The greatest numbers of soil-transmitted helminth infections occur in sub-Saharan Africa, the Americas, China and east Asia.

Infection is caused by ingestion of eggs from contaminated soil (*Ascaris lumbricoides* and *Trichuris trichiura*) or by active penetration of the skin by larvae in the soil (hookworms).

Soil-transmitted helminths produce a wide range of symptoms that include intestinal manifestations (diarrhoea, abdominal pain), general malaise and weakness that may affect working and learning capacities, and impaired physical growth. Hookworms cause chronic intestinal blood loss that results in anaemia.

Recommended intervention strategy and aim

Targeted administration of albendazole, mebendazole, levamisole or pyrantel. The frequency of intervention is determined by the levels of prevalence of infection among school-age children (see Annex 2). The aim is morbidity control: periodic treatment of at-risk populations will reduce the intensity of infection and protect infected individuals from morbidity due to soil-transmitted helminthiasis.

Eligible population

Preschool and school-age children, women of childbearing age (including pregnant women in the 2nd and 3rd trimesters and lactating women), and adults at high risk in certain occupations (e.g. tea-pickers and miners).

Ineligible population

Children in the 1st year of life; pregnant women in the 1st trimester of pregnancy.

Access to drugs

Where the drugs are not donated, the average market price of a single tablet of generic albendazole or mebendazole is around US$ 0.02–0.03.

World Health Assembly targets and deadlines

Resolution WHA54.19 (2001) urged Member States "…to ensure access to essential drugs against…soil-transmitted helminth infections in all health services in endemic areas for the treatment of clinical cases and groups at high risk of morbidity such as women and children, with the goal of attaining a minimum target of regular administration of chemotherapy to at least 75% and up to 100% of all school-age children at risk of morbidity by 2010".

Web site

http://www.who.int/neglected_diseases/diseases/en/

---

[1] Crompton DWT & Savioli L. 2006. Handbook of Helminthiasis for Public Health. Boca Raton, Florida - Taylor and Francis Group, LLC.

Lymphatic filariasis

- *Operational guidelines for rapid mapping of bancroftian filariasis in Africa.* Geneva, World Health Organization, 2000 (WHO/CDS/CPE/CEE/2000.9).
- *Training module on community home-based prevention of disability due to lymphatic filariasis.* Geneva, World Health Organization, 2003 (WHO/CDS/CPE/CEE/2003.35).
- *Lymphatic filariasis elimination programme: training module for drug distributors in areas where lymphatic filariasis is not co-endemic with onchocerciasis.* Geneva, World Health Organization (WHO/CDS/CPE/CEE/2001.22).
- *Lymphatic filariasis elimination programme: training module for drug distributors in areas where lymphatic filariasis is co-endemic with onchocerciasis.* Geneva, World Health Organization, 2004 (WHO/CDS/CPE/CEE/2001.23).
- *Monitoring and epidemiological assessment of the programme to eliminate lymphatic filariasis at implementation unit level.* Geneva, World Health Organization, 2005 (WHO/CDS/CPE/CEE/2005.50).

Onchocerciasis

- Ngoumou P & Walsh JF. *A manual for rapid epidemiological mapping of onchocerciasis.* Geneva, World Health Organization, 1993 (TDR/TDE/ONCHO/93.4).
- *Onchocerciasis and its control. Report of a WHO Expert Committee on Onchocerciasis Control.* Geneva, World Health Organization, 1995 (WHO Technical Report Series, No. 852).
- *Certification of elimination of human onchocerciasis: criteria and procedures.* Geneva, World Health Organization, 2001 (WHO/CDS/CPE/CEE/2001.18a).

Schistosomiasis and soil-transmitted helminths

- Montresor A et al. *Helminth control in school-age children: a guide for managers of control programmes.* Geneva, World Health Organization, 2002.
- *Prevention and control of schistosomiasis and soil-transmitted helminthiasis. Report of a WHO Expert Committee.* Geneva, World Health Organization, 2002 (WHO Technical Report Series, No. 912).
- *Report on the WHO Informal Consultation on the use of praziquantel during pregnancy/lactation and albendazole/mebendazole in children under 24 months.* Geneva, World Health Organization, 2003 (WHO/CDS/CPE/PVC/2002.4).
- *How to add deworming to vitamin A distribution.* Geneva, World Health Organization, 2004 (WHO/CDS/CPE/PVC/2004.11).

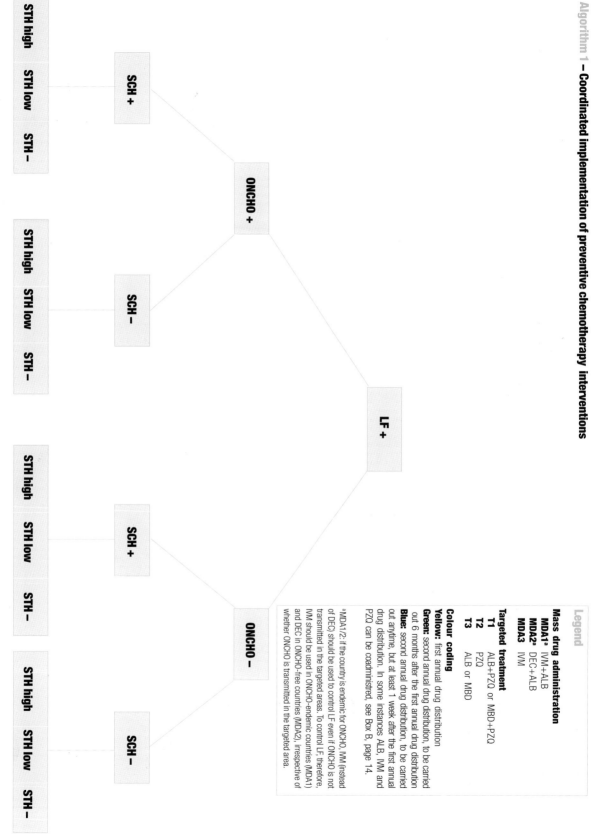

Algorithm 1 – Coordinated implementation of preventive chemotherapy interventions

ONCHO +
- SCH +
  - STH high — MDA1 T1
  - STH low — MDA1 T2
  - STH − — MDA1 T2
- SCH −
  - STH high — MDA1 T3
  - STH low — MDA1
  - STH − — MDA1

LF +
- ONCHO +
- ONCHO −
  - SCH +
    - STH high — MDA1/2ᵃ T1
    - STH low — MDA1/2 T2
    - STH − — MDA1/2 T2
  - SCH −
    - STH high — MDA1/2ᵃ T3
    - STH low — MDA1/2ᵃ
    - STH − — MDA1/2ᵃ

Legend

Mass drug administration
- **MDA1ᵃ** IVM+ALB
- **MDA2ᵃ** DEC+ALB
- **MDA3** IVM

Targeted treatment
- **T1** ALB+PZQ or MBD+PZQ
- **T2** PZQ
- **T3** ALB or MBD

Colour coding
- **Yellow:** first annual drug distribution
- **Green:** second annual drug distribution, to be carried out 6 months after the first annual drug distribution
- **Blue:** second annual drug distribution, to be carried out anytime, but at least 1 week after the first annual drug distribution. In some instances ALB, IVM and PZQ can be coadministered, see Box B, page 14.

ᵃ MDA1/2: if the country is endemic for ONCHO, IVM (instead of DEC) should be used to control LF even if ONCHO is not transmitted in the targeted areas. To control LF, therefore, IVM should be used in ONCHO-endemic countries (MDA1) and DEC in ONCHO-free countries (MDA2), irrespective of whether ONCHO is transmitted in the targeted area.

Algorithm 2 – Coordinated implementation of preventive chemotherapy interventions

Decision tree structure:

- **LF –**
  - **ONCHO +**
    - **SCH +**
      - STH high → MDA1 T1
      - STH low → MDA1 T2
      - STH – → MDA3 T2
    - **SCH –**
      - STH high → MDA1 T3
      - STH low → MDA1
      - STH – → MDA3
  - **ONCHO –**
    - **SCH +**
      - STH high → T1 T3
      - STH low → T1
      - STH – → T2
    - **SCH –**
      - STH high → T3 T3
      - STH low → T3
      - STH – → No action required

Form 1: for village/urban area/school/health post recording of drug coverage (MDA1, MDA2, MDA3)

Region:			Village/urban area/school/health post:	
District:			Campaign/round of treatment:	
Date:			Drugs distributed:	

Class/household/ treatment point	Total population	Eligible population	Number of individuals ingesting an appropriate dose of treatment [cross out the ALB column in MDA3 interventions]	
			ALB	IVM/DEC
1				
2				
3				
4				
5				
6				
7				
8				
9				
10				
11				
12				
13				
14				
15				
16				
17				
18				
19				
20				
21				
22				
23				
24				
25				
26				
27				
28				
29				
30				

Total by village/urban area/school/health post:

Village/ urban area/ school/ health post	(A) Total population	(B) Eligible population	No. of individuals ingesting an appropriate dose of treatment:		Reported coverage	
			(C) ALB	(D) IVM/DEC	% of total population $(D/A) \times 100$	% of eligible population $(D/B) \times 100$

Form 2: for district reporting of drug coverage (MDA1, MDA2, MDA3)

Region:			Campaign/round of treatment:			
District:			Campaign/round of treatment:			
Date:			Drugs distributed:			
Total number of urban areas in district:			Total number of villages in district:			
Number of urban areas covered:			Number of villages covered:			

Village/ urban area/ school/ health post	Targeted for ONCHO (Y/N)	Total population	Eligible population	Number of individuals ingesting an appropriate dose of treatment [cross out the ALB column in MDA3 interventions]		Reported drug coverage	
				ALB	IVM/DEC	% of total population	% of eligible population
1							
2							
3							
4							
5							
6							
7							
8							
9							
10							
11							
12							
13							
14							
15							
16							
17							
18							
19							
20							
21							
22							
23							
24							
25							
26							
27							
28							
29							
30							

Total by district:							
District		(A) Total population	(B) Eligible population	Number of individuals ingesting an appropriate dose of treatment		Reported coverage	
				(C) ALB	(D) IVM/DEC	% of total population (D/A) x 100	% of eligible population (D/B) x 100

Form 3: for village/urban area/school/health post recording of drug coverage (T1, T2, T3)

Region:		Village/urban area/school/health post:	
District:		Campaign/round of treatment:	
Date:		Drugs distributed:	

Class/ household/ treatment point	Number of eligible individuals	Number of targeted individuals	Number of targeted individuals ingesting an appropriate dose of treatment: [cross out the ALB/MBD column in T2 interventions; cross out the PZQ column in T3 interventions]	
			ALB/MBD	PZQ
1				
2				
3				
4				
5				
6				
7				
8				
9				
10				
11				
12				
13				
14				
15				
16				
17				
18				
19				
20				
21				
22				
23				
24				
25				
26				
27				
28				
29				
30				

Total by village/urban area/school/health post:

Village/urban area/school/ health post	Number of eligible individuals	Number of targeted individuals	Number of targeted individuals ingesting an appropriate dose of treatment		Coverage (%)
			ALB/MBD	PZQ	

Form 4: for district recording of drug coverage (T1, T2, T3)

Region:		Campaign/round of treatment:	
District:			
Date:		Drugs distributed:	

Village/ urban area/ school/ health post	Number of targeted individuals	Number of targeted individuals ingesting an appropriate dose of treatment: [cross out the ALB/MBD column in T2 interventions; cross out the PZQ column in T3 interventions		Coverage (%)
		ALB/MBD	PZQ	
1				
2				
3				
4				
5				
6				
7				
8				
9				
10				
11				
12				
13				
14				
15				
16				
17				
18				
19				
20				
21				
22				
23				
24				
25				
26				
27				
28				
29				
30				

Total by district:

District	Number of targeted individuals	Number of targeted individuals receiving an appropriate dose of treatment		Coverage %
		ALB/MBD	PZQ